Stepping
Out

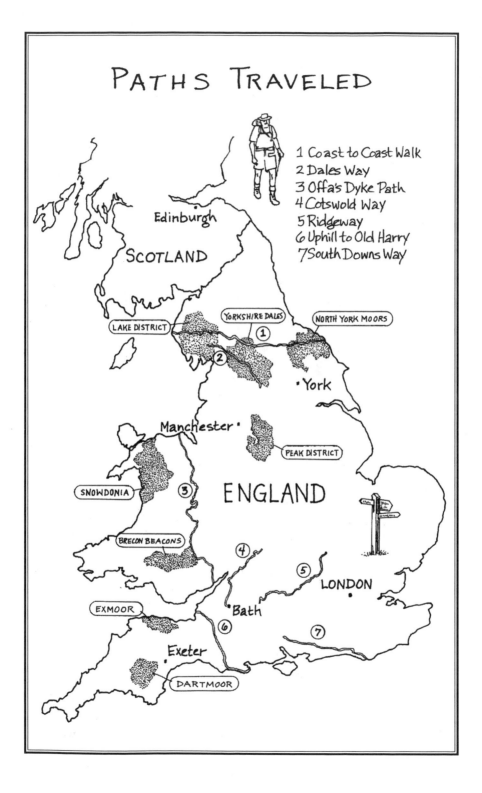

PATHS TRAVELED

1 Coast to Coast Walk
2 Dales Way
3 Offa's Dyke Path
4 Cotswold Way
5 Ridgeway
6 Uphill to Old Harry
7 South Downs Way

SCOTLAND

Edinburgh

ENGLAND

LAKE DISTRICT

YORKSHIRE DALES

NORTH YORK MOORS

York

Manchester

PEAK DISTRICT

SNOWDONIA

BRECON BEACONS

LONDON

Bath

EXMOOR

Exeter

DARTMOOR

Stepping Out

A Tenderfoot's Guide to the Principles, Practices, and Pleasures of Countryside Walking

Eleanor Garrell Berger

Tenderfoot Press
Plattsburgh, New York

Tenderfoot Press, LLC
Plattsburgh, NY
www.tenderfootpress.com

Stepping Out has been written for the pleasure of the reader. The book is not intended to provide professional advice on health or fitness. The author and publisher urge readers to use sound judgment and care while enjoying the recreational activities described and to consult a medical professional before attempting any new physical exercise. The author discusses appropriate clothing and equipment but does not endorse any products or services. *Stepping Out* is not a trail guide. Readers should refer to up-to-date guidebooks and websites for information about specific walks and trails.

The author is grateful for permission to reprint a quotation from the *South Downs Way* – National Trail Guide by Paul Millmore, published by Aurum Press, Ltd.

Printed in the United States of America

ISBN: 978-0-9816475-0-0
Library of Congress Control Number: 2008924249

Designed by Sara Kurak
Cover art and illustrations by Elayne Sears

Dedication

For every tenderfoot who says, "I'll try."

For all who cherish the countryside and walk its footpaths.

For my parents, Louis and Lillian Garrell,
my first and best writing teachers.

And for Mike, who makes dreams come true.

Contents

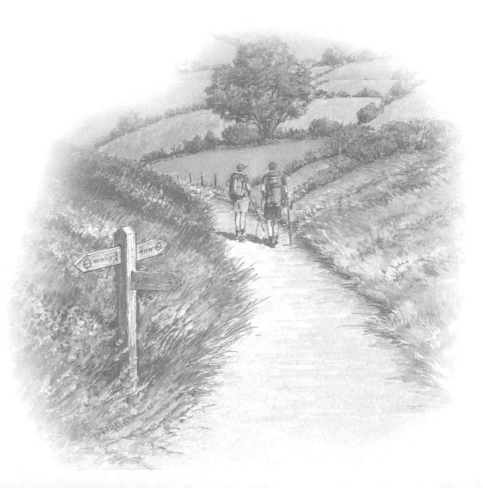

Acknowledgments

First, I thank my partner, Michael DiNunzio, wonderful person and outstanding walking companion, for reducing my excuses to procrastinate by his walking dogs, shoveling snow, and making meals. I also thank him for his insights, suggestions, and edits, and for believing in me when I did not believe in myself.

Next, I thank the members of my creative publishing team for their "we-can-do-it" spirit, their friendship, and for their optimism when deadlines loomed. I thank Sheila J. Levine for her legal advice, personal assurances, and Sunday phone calls; Holly Crawford for her magic red pen, her gentle (but frank) corrections, and her attention to detail; Sara Kurak for making my words look good and for introducing me to possibility; Elayne Sears for turning ideas into charming images and for doing so with a smile; Gary Lambert, computer and website guru, for solving digital dilemmas and calming my electronic fears; and Kathy Archer for lifting the curtain on publicity and getting this book and me out and about.

I especially thank Paul Millmore for introducing Mike and me to countryside walking. I thank him for his guidance and hospitality, for listening and teaching, for editing and making me laugh, and for always saying "yes." I also thank Bridget Millmore for hosting and nourishing Mike and me and for providing us with company and sustenance on the last day of our last walk.

I thank Robert and JoAnne Withington, walking mentors and friends, for their advice, support, and empathy. I thank Diane Wiltjer for telling me to write this book, and Ed and Maureen Gardner for their dedication to outfitting a tenderfoot. I thank and hug Cathy Frank for sharing, commiserating, and building confidence. I thank—and thank again—my first and final manuscript reader and lifelong, loving friend, Tina Kostecki Califano, for always being with me, even from afar.

I thank the people who have expanded my writing life: Michael McGaulley, author of *The Grail Conspiracies*, for his coaching and suggestions; Allen and Linda Anderson of Angel Animals Network; Mary Carpenter, editor of *Plattsburgh Alive*; Laurel Lloyd Earnshaw and Pat Johnson, editors of *Aurora*; the wonderful people at North Country Public Radio, and at Northeast Public Radio; and the late Judi Sklar Becker, editor of *Good Dog! Magazine*. I especially want to thank the remarkable Nancy Slonim Aronie, author of *Writing from the Heart*, and teacher extraordinaire, for giving me wings and persuading me that I could soar.

I thank Kellie Rowden-Racette for making research look easy and Sharon Banhold for uncovering the obscure. I thank Mary Paul, Jessica Jarvis, Elsie Jarvis, and Joan Kogut for taking care of our precious dogs and things at home while Mike and I traveled.

I thank the many generous and enthusiastic citizens in my Plattsburgh community for cheering on my literary efforts: Sharon Boice for her humor and perspective; Ashley Moore for her expert photocopying and for listening; William W. Drew, for his forbearance and mastery of numbers; Sandra Walker for her support and assistance; and all the good and helpful people at my local bank, post office, League of Women Voters, Sisterhood, and Rotary Club.

For their encouragement, I thank the finest friends in the world: Lenore Forsted, Sonia Long, and Carole Slatkin for their candid comments and useful suggestions; and Bunny Adler, Carole Berger, Jo Ann Hewett, Shelby Berger Jakoby, Nancy Perry, and Sara Rowden for their sustained support.

I am indebted to the Berger family for wonderful memories and a lifetime of generosity. My gratitude also goes to my terrific bothers, Martin Garrell and Howard Garrell, and to my astute sister-in-law, Janet Garrell.

I am grateful beyond measure to friends in the UK, whom Mike and I first met on our Coast to Coast Walk. They continue to walk with us in many ways. Thank you to Colin Lawson for joining us on the Cotswold Way and, again, with his wife, Liz, to celebrate our completing the Ridgeway walk. Thank you to David and Sheila Gale for sharing our tales of adventure, offering splendid advice, driving hours to spend evenings with us at bed and breakfasts on our footpaths, and showing us a bit of Wales on a rainy day. Thank you to Mike and Margaret Fagg and their dog Poppy for joining us on three walks with maps in hand, humor intact, bird and flower guides at the ready, and Scottish shortbread in their packs.

I send a countryside full of gratitude to Robin and Joan Loveday for giving Mike and me many reasons to smile. Thank you to Joan for being an elegant hostess and for taking part in our walks, most recently by telephone or in person at dinners along the way. I extend my deepest gratitude to Robin, who has walked six hundred miles with us, carrying a phone, GPS unit, maps, and a trail guide. We thank Robin for his wonderful stories, optimistic outlook, and good nature—and for helping to make every mile of our walks together a delight.

Finally, to those who work and campaign to make countryside walking the pleasure it is, and to all the charming, funny, curious ramblers we have met along the way, thank you. Thank you so very much.

"I only went out for a walk,
and finally concluded to stay out till sundown,
for going out, I found, was really going in."

John Muir (1838–1914)
My First Summer in the Sierra (1911)

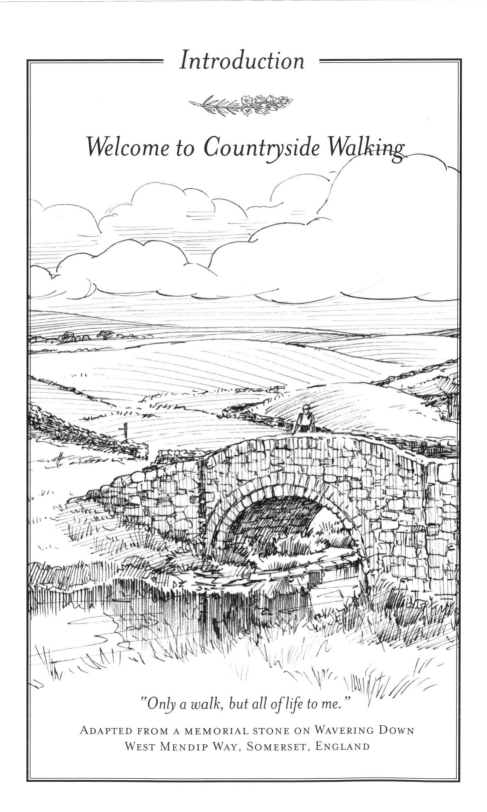

Welcome to Countryside Walking

"Only a walk, but all of life to me."

ADAPTED FROM A MEMORIAL STONE ON WAVERING DOWN
WEST MENDIP WAY, SOMERSET, ENGLAND

Dear Tenderfoot

THIS BOOK *is* FOR YOU, IF YOU...
- enjoy walking
- prefer country paths to sidewalks and roads
- think you might like to walk for several days
- can't decide what to wear or pack for a week or more of rambling
- like to stay at bed and breakfasts and small inns
- enjoy visiting new places, eating unfamiliar food, and having fun off the beaten track
- want to improve your health with pleasant outdoor exercise

THIS BOOK *is not* FOR YOU, IF YOU...
- are unable to slow down
- like your sports extreme
- are considering a technical climb in the Himalayas
- prefer bushwhacking through wilderness to walking on well-trodden paths
- welcome the challenge of digging your own latrine
- enjoy discomfort and inconvenience

An Invitation

On most Saturdays in the spring, after the snow melts and the mud hardens, Mike and I leash our dog for a family outing at a local park. A walk in the fresh air is our escape from an ever-expanding list of responsibilities. And, as my mother liked to say, "A nice walk puts color in your cheeks."

On one outing, obviously intoxicated by an abundance of oxygen and enthusiasm, I felt inspiration overcome inhibition. "Wouldn't it be fun," I wondered aloud, "if we could walk a little further, explore a less familiar trail, and arrive at a place more inviting than a parking lot?" This was an odd thought for a tenderfoot like me.

Dedicated as I am to avoiding the challenges of discomfort, I prefer to confine my quests for adventure to books and movies about rescues at sea and survival at high altitudes. I marvel at the audacity of foreign correspondents, assigned to dangerous, dusty places, and cannot imagine packing for Kabul in a carry-on or traveling to Kinshasa without my hair dryer.

Yet, one year after voicing my uncharacteristic inspiration, I was walking in the English countryside—a pack on my back, my hair dryer abandoned—looking forward to a pub dinner, a night under a cozy duvet, a full English breakfast, and another day of rambling across the South Downs. This is the story of how such miracles happen and how they can happen for you.

Countryside walking is not for those who dream of hiking to Everest Base Camp or sailing single-handedly around the world. Much gentler than that, it is an un-extreme form of adventure, perfect for those of us who prefer slower, less taxing travel along pleasant paths of discovery and awareness.

I wrote *Stepping Out* to introduce the hesitant adventurer to the delights of countryside walking, to entice the daily walker to set off on a long-distance footpath, and to share familiar pleasures with the committed rambler. Its pages are filled with anecdotes, journal entries, personal essays, instructive tips, and practical advice about traveling comfortably across the countryside on one's own two feet.

Stepping Out combines my passion for giving advice with my love of rambling. Its message is simple: *You can do it.* You can trek up hill and down dale. You can carry a light pack, walk in the rain, and have a wonderful, guiltless time eating all you want. And every day, as you move forward to your next lodging, feeling proud and courageous, you will grow stronger in many ways.

So, reach for your walking stick, step out of your comfort zone, and join me for a gentle walk in the countryside. It's time to put some color in our cheeks.

How to Use This Book

Stepping Out can be read in any order. Skim or savor its essays and advice, in or out of sequence. Begin with the "how to" hints in its early chapters or the detailed information in Step Fourteen to help you prepare for and plan your adventure. Or read these fact-filled chapters later. You might even skip them entirely if you're already familiar with what to buy, how to pack, and how to plan a walking itinerary.

Perhaps you'll begin with one of the chapters that describes what it's like to follow a footpath, sleep in a different bed almost every night, eat in a pub, walk in the rain, or reach the end of a trail.

Chapters contain a mixture of observations, facts, memories, and vignettes gathered over many years, while Mike and I were planning long-distance walks and day trips, and rambling along hundreds of miles of footpaths. (For more about specific trails, see "Paths Taken" in Step Fourteen.) Sample a few pages, or read them all, as you uncover the principles, practices, and pleasures of countryside walking.

The way you read *Stepping Out* is not important. What matters is that you enjoy every step of your journey as we walk along together.

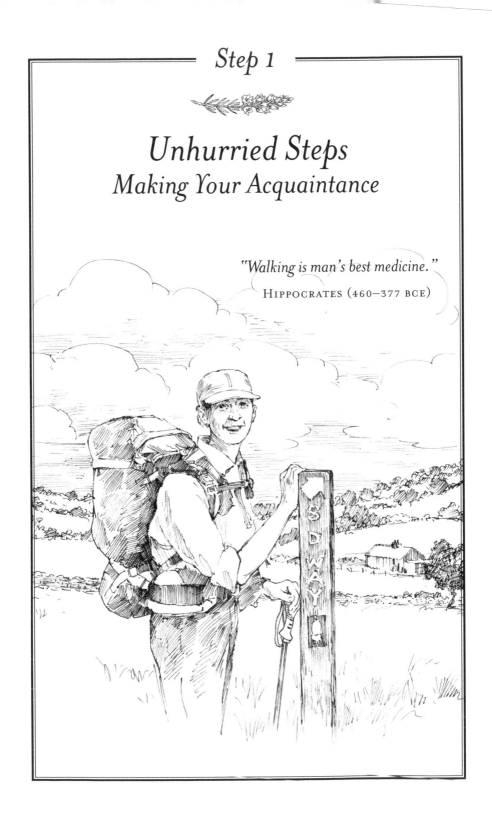

Unhurried Steps
Making Your Acquaintance

"Walking is man's best medicine."

Hippocrates (460–377 BCE)

First Person Present

Not Me

Pleasure, Not Pain

Walking One Hundred Miles
    Journal: Just Right

Perfect Setting

Answers Please

The Company We Keep

Definitions
A Tenderfoot
Good Walking Companions
Country Walkers
Forms of Locomotion
    Climbing
    Hiking or Backpacking
    Trekking
    Rambling or Tramping
    Walking

First Person Present

I've spent most of my life—and all of my college years—trying to figure out who I am. I'm still not sure. Answers keep shifting with age, slipping from my grasp. But since we'll be walking together, I'd like to tell you who I think I am at the moment. And, more important, who I'm not and probably never will be.

I was born a "what-if" person. I matured into a "what-if" traveler, which is why I feel compelled to pack for contingencies: what if it rains, what if it's cold, what if I cut myself, twist an ankle, rip my luggage? I aspire to become a "what-me-worry" individual, but so far, no go. Whether readying for a short trip or a long walk, packing for me is a major undertaking because I want to carry *everything* I think I might need.

I was reared in New York City in a loving but "indoorsy" family. A trip to the Prospect Park Zoo, a day exploring exotica at the Brooklyn Botanic Garden, or a ride on a bumper car at Coney Island passed for outdoor expeditions. Strenuous activity meant punch ball in the school yard, hopscotch or potsy on a chalked sidewalk, or roller skating on four sensible, "out-of-line" wheels. I walked everywhere, but not too energetically. Exertion was alien behavior. I don't remember ever sweating in PE.

In college I loved geology classes. I was fascinated with the ways in which rocks explained the physical world. I planned to major in the subject, but switched to political science when I discovered that geology majors had to spend part of the summer after their junior year camped out somewhere on the Colorado Plateau—an impossibility for a tenderfoot.

I married a few days out of college and wanted very much to please my new husband, who liked to ski and loved to sail. I did both somewhat reluctantly, with as much good sportsmanship as a warm weather skier and a fair-weather sailor could muster—which was not enough for me to really embrace outdoor recreation. My late husband should be sainted for teaching me to sail, as should all those ski instructors who endured my attempts to master the parallel turn. I had fun outdoors, but not as much fun as I had indoors at concerts, restaurants, theaters, and dance classes.

I loved to travel, as long as I could do so in comfort. I pouted a lot when I couldn't. Occasionally, I would step out of my comfort niche to enjoy a bit of adventure on a tour in some wild and wonderful land and was almost always happy that I had.

Recently, I discovered that I loved walking, especially with another person along to share the experience. This is why the idea of walking a little further in pleasant surroundings with a companion beckoned me, and why my new life partner, Mike, and I decided to venture beyond our local park.

What I didn't realize was that walking for several days in a lovely countryside setting would set me on a path of personal discovery; that sustained physical activity would soon change, not just who I was, but who I might become; and that, along the way, I would have the time of my life.

Not Me

I am not an athlete, although I do walk one to three miles almost every day, mostly because I have a dog that requires outings. I'm also the designated hunter/gatherer/schlepper of household goods and groceries.

Among my dear friends, however, I count five athletic women. So it's easy to observe that, as active as I am, "athletic" I am not. For example, I'm not Leslie. Leslie is rugged. Her idea of fun is one hundred miles of cycling across the Midwest by day, sleeping in school gymnasiums at night. I'm not Sara, either, whose favorite activities at the moment include flinging her body through space on a trapeze and careening downhill on a snowboard. Nor am I a serious hiker like Cathy, who last summer hiked the Long Trail in Vermont, spending her days on rocky mountain slopes and her evenings cooking out, sharing a lean-to with strangers, and loving it.

I am certainly not "Belt Woman," that skinny-Minnie in a tool belt bikini, who renovates bathrooms and replaces ceilings on TV home improvement shows. Capable and confident, she is perpetually pleasant. Of course, I would be, too, if I could complete major projects in fewer than thirty minutes. Belt Woman never panics or cries when things go wrong. In her life, they seldom do.

We tender-footed souls may not be as athletic or as mechanically competent as our friends, but if we step out, beyond the limits of who we think we are, some day even *we* may evolve into stronger, braver, and more able beings, willing to strap on a tool belt or swing from a trapeze. Some day, perhaps, but not yet. Which is why a long walk in a lovely setting is a perfect choice for us.

Pleasure, Not Pain

Be assured: countryside walking is always pleasurable, although perhaps a bit less so on a rainy, cold, muddy day. Even then, it is never punitive.

A punitive vacation is the kind my friend Anna prefers. It is her idea of fun. She thrives on discomfort, overdoses on challenge, and carries good sportsmanship to an extreme. She races down rapids, scrambles up rocky overhangs, and treks at high altitudes. One year she bicycled around the world. Hers is precisely the type of travel a tenderfoot avoids.

Exactly how does one go about biking around the world? How does one pack and shop? How does one locate medical attention in a remote village? What does one do if one's bike falls apart? It's all too much to imagine, too stressful even to contemplate.

And yet, Anna's spirit of adventure lives in every soul—even mine. For me, however, a long walk is adventure enough. I prefer to leave "punitive" holidays to others.

Walking One Hundred Miles

When you begin planning a long walk, everyone you tell about it will ask six questions—the same six questions—over and over. The first five are easy:

- How far are you planning to walk?
- How many days will that take you?
- How much are you going to carry?
- Where will you stay at night?
- What will you do if it rains?

The sixth question is the tough one: Why are you doing this? Translation: Why in the world would anyone want to walk one hundred miles or more?

"Well," you might answer, "Why wouldn't I want to take a long walk in an interesting location? Walking is fun. It's natural. And I've been doing it all my life."

A more helpful answer, however, might resemble one I wrote in my journal to address my own concerns before our first journey.

━━━━━━━━━━ ❦ J o u r n a l ━

Just Right

I want to sample local landscapes and the charms of village life. I want to replace traffic, neon, and plastic with natural, unhurried spaces. I want to move forward on my own two feet and see if I like doing it in muddy boots.

I don't want to conquer anything, except my own reluctance. I want to push myself, but not too much. Like Goldilocks, I want something that is "just right" for me. Wilderness camping and mountain trekking are too hard. Walks around the block are too soft. But a journey of eight to ten miles per day? That could be "just right," especially if each day ends at a bed and breakfast with a warm welcome, clean sheets, and hot water.

I want to learn to live with less. I don't know yet what "less" is for ten days of walking or whether it will fit into a pack I can carry. I would like to keep all my belongings with me on my back, rather than in a duffel bag for sending ahead. I want to discover if I can leave behind my "large suitcase life" and find happiness in a light backpack.

I want to challenge myself without overtaxing my spirit with more discomfort than I can handle. I know that I whine when I'm cold, I complain when I'm tired, and I grumble when I'm hungry. What I don't know is whether I can be a good sport on a rainy day when my feet hurt.

I want to share an adventure with people on whom I can depend. I want to be brave. I want to do something different (but civilized) in a place that is new to me. And I want to enjoy the experience.

I have never done anything like this before; I'm not sure I can do it now. Sometimes I wonder why I even want to try. 🖾

Perfect Setting

Beautiful walking is everywhere: Tuscany and Provence, New Zealand and Vermont, Nepal and Bhutan. We made our decision about where we would go on our walk when friends invited us to stay with them in southern England. It was from their home that our first journey of one hundred miles began. A bit of reading as our plans got underway revealed that we had, quite literally, stumbled onto some of the finest walking paths on earth.

Walking in Britain is world class. Rambling, in fact, is a national pastime—and with good reason. A walker can enjoy a scenic, short stroll, carrying only a day pack, or opt for the challenge of walking a week or more over longer distances.

With thousands of miles of off-road public paths, there is something for everyone: valley walks and high peak trails, towpaths and riverside footpaths, woodland and farm tracks, and country and village lanes. Trails wind through thousands of acres of public forest and across open tracts, many of which are owned by the National Trust, as well as by individual landowners.

Many British walks are journeys through history. Paths that attract today's ramblers may be centuries old. Some follow medieval tracks. Others follow parts of roads built during four hundred years of Roman occupation, beginning in the first century.

Public access to vast stretches of private, working landscape throughout the countryside expands the pleasure of walking. Since people live and farm along the footpaths, visitors can stay in farmhouses, cottages, hostels, inns, and homes on estates, meeting local people and making new friends. With sleeping accommodations and pubs so numerous and varied along a trail, walkers can adjust the distances they travel each day. For all these reasons—and more—Britain has become a favorite destination for those who like to trek, tramp, and ramble across the countryside.

Answers Please
Questions to Consider before Stepping Out

- How many days do I wish to walk?
- How fit am I?
- How may hours each day do I want to walk?
- How many miles will I average each day?
- What kind of terrain can I manage?
- What are my favorite outdoor temperatures for walking?

  Note: A great countryside walk for me—someone who walks one to three miles on local streets about five days a week—is eight to twelve miles a day on easy-to-moderate terrain for seven to ten days. I feel happiest in fall-like weather with dry trails under foot and sunshine over head. Unfortunately, I have yet to discover how to ensure such ideal conditions.

- Do I wish to walk alone, with a companion, in a group of old friends, or on a tour with new friends?
- Do I want to make my own plans, work with an agent to arrange a self-guided tour, or find a preplanned walking tour that suits me?
- Do I prefer to stay in a cozy spot and enjoy day walks, or would I like to follow a trail, staying in a new location each night?
- Do I prefer walking in and around cities? Would I like to visit farms, villages, and historic sites, or explore wilder, remote, natural areas?
- Do I like following marked trails? Can I read a map or use a GPS unit?

  Note: With trail guides, waymarks, and people to ask, walkers can get around without getting seriously lost.

- Can I manage a whole day in the great outdoors without modern conveniences?

  Note: If you have never answered nature's call "al fresco," be assured that doing so is easy and liberating. (Look for some helpful hints in Step Ten.)

- Will I be happy with all my belongings on my back, or would I rather carry a day pack and send my luggage on ahead?

  Note: My partner Mike and I prefer to carry our belongings—about 23 pounds of them—on our backs. But, as we grow a bit longer in the tooth and weaker in the knee, the idea of sending our belongings ahead with a luggage service and carrying only a light day pack is gaining appeal.

The Company We Keep

Mike, with whom I have been traveling through life for almost two decades, is also my walking companion. I'm fortunate to have found in one person someone who fills both roles.

This is not to imply that we are entirely compatible. When I opted for a group tour to Alaska, I went with my friend Anne. If I go to the ballet, I go with Sonia. I visit museums with Carole, concerts with Nancy, and dog shows with Janet. Mike prefers his adventures outdoors, close to nature.

Over lunch, on our first date, I felt compelled to tell him, "I'm not rugged," "I don't do 'cold and wet' very well because they make me grumpy," and "I'm far better at 'civilized and comfortable.'"

I placed my confession on the table, along with our salads, the minute after Mike told me that back in the seventies he walked the entire Appalachian Trail—over two thousand miles of it—in a five-and-a-half-month period. He assured me that this kind of escapade was out of his system, but I was reluctant to accept first date assurances.

He was being honest, however. Having "been there, done that," he hikes now with a day pack for his own pleasure and spiritual renewal, not to prove or to conquer anything. In nice weather, I hike with him—not too far and not too fast, but enough to appreciate that being outside enhances one's "inside" and that nature does good things for one's soul.

Unless you prefer to walk alone, choosing a companion is the first and most important decision you will make. Group tours offer some security because they provide a selection of companions for walking, dining, and conversation. Putting together your own group of friends, or choosing just one companion as I did, requires a bit more care.

Bear in mind that walking together over several days is not like going to the opera where, if your companion doesn't like the performance, he'll only be unhappy for a few hours, which he can spend inside a warm and comfortable theater where he has choices. He can relax in the lobby, visit a clean rest room, or leave and meet you somewhere later. On a footpath, choices are limited.

If you're not walking with a group and don't wish to walk alone, look for a companion who believes you will reach whatever destination you've set your heart on. Find someone who laughs easily and is not bothered by rain or mediocre restaurant service; who is silly, reliable, and considerate; who is patient, easy-going, and enthusiastic; and who is more surefooted than you are. In short, choose a friend—or someone you'd like to have for a friend.

Definitions

A TENDERFOOT
- Can walk a few miles a day several days a week
- Chooses adventure that is safe and enjoyable
- Likes physical challenge, but not discomfort
- Thinks about *stepping out* beyond the familiar and predictable into a bold, fresh identity
- Is ready, willing, and able (but reluctant) to go on a countryside walk

GOOD WALKING COMPANIONS
- Can cope with you when you're barely coping
- Can view a crisis as a situation
- Can be nice when they're tired or hungry
- Can read a trail map or use a GPS unit
- Can pack light
- Are in condition for walking
- Are good sports
- Are not fussy eaters
- Don't disturb your sleep with snoring
- Enjoy conversation
- Think you are special

Country Walkers

- *Enjoy* walking, smiling, making new friends, and seeing new places "up close and personal"; observing and photographing nature and village life; and eating with gusto
- *Want to* improve their fitness, boost their energy, lower their stress, improve their health, tone their muscles, clear their minds, and sharpen their senses—all while engaging in adventure that is relaxing, refreshing, and fun
- *Like* leaving the predictable and familiar behind to visit new places
- *Know* that there will never be a better time to get started, and that they don't have to finish a walk to feel elated, but that finishing is deeply satisfying

Forms of Locomotion

What will you be doing once you're on your feet and underway? The answer is confusing because many walking terms are used interchangeably, but not consistently. Below are some of my own definitions for common forms of bipedal forward motion and the ones I will use in this book.

Climbing (Very Difficult)

What you do when you struggle upward and, perhaps, rappel downward. This requires using your hands occasionally and following questionable trails that have a way of getting washed out. Not recommended for a tenderfoot.

Hiking or Backpacking (Difficult)

Hardy walking with a good bit of slogging, usually followed by a night in a tent or lean-to and a dinner of rehydrated food at a campsite without running water. Not a first choice for a tenderfoot.

Trekking (Moderate)

A long, often strenuous, walk of more than about fifty miles over several days that includes some steep hills. A tenderfoot who is fit and pain free will enjoy trekking and will feel pleasantly tired at day's end. *Note: In the Himalayas, all walks, even easy ones, are referred to as "treks."*

Rambling or Tramping (Easy to Moderate)

The splendid, total experience of moving under one's own power across the countryside. A ramble is a sustained walk with a purpose. It's what walkers, absorbed by their surroundings, are doing as they head toward a welcome destination. It clears the mind and frees the soul. Rambling brings joy and well-being to the tenderfoot and to just about everyone else.

Walking (Easy to Moderate)

A memorable, multipurpose activity enjoyed by millions. All rambles are walks, although the reverse may not be true. A tenderfoot gets ready for rambling or trekking by walking. In the States, where our landscape has been chopped up and paved over to accommodate the automobile and suburban sprawl, we have pleasant neighborhoods for walking, but very few off-road paths for long rambles. Walking is pleasurable for the tenderfoot and athlete alike, as daily exercise or as the focus of a vacation.

Note: It doesn't really matter how you define what you're doing, except in Britain, where it's best to refer to yourself as a "walker" or a "rambler" when you reserve a room. If you say you're a "hiker," you might be considered a bit too dirty and rough for indoor accommodations and may not be welcome at a proper B & B. So whether you're on a trek or a ramble, identify yourself as a "walker," which is a mighty fine thing to be.

Step 2

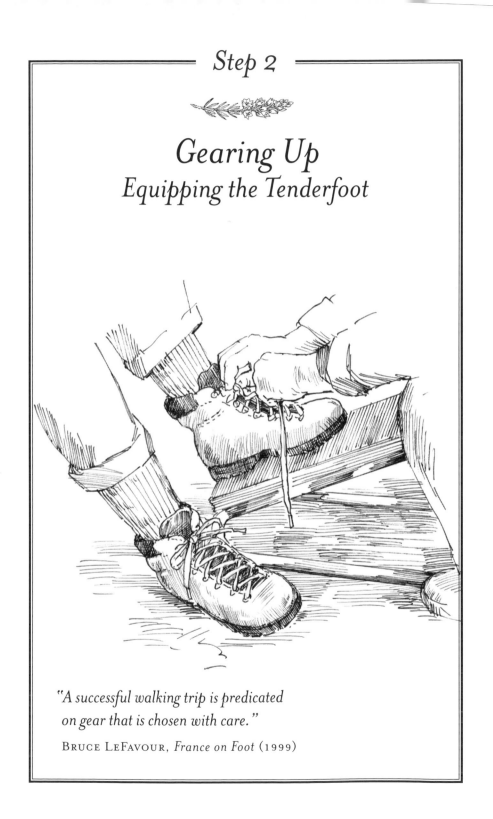

Gearing Up
Equipping the Tenderfoot

*"A successful walking trip is predicated
on gear that is chosen with care."*

BRUCE LEFAVOUR, *France on Foot* (1999)

Getting Familiar

Walking Sticks (Poles)

Shopping

Moving On

Feet never feel as tired walking a hundred–mile
footpath as they do treading the retail trail.

Step Two of our walking adventure requires a bit of hunting and gathering, which is why you won't want to leave "gearing up" for the last minute. By starting early, you'll avoid racing through stores and scavenging
through closets, increasing your stress and reducing your fun, just before
departure. So give yourself plenty of time to locate what you need and to
return and exchange what you don't. After you've acquired and shaken
down your essentials, future journeys can be rapid, pack-and-go kinds of
affairs. But your first walk, which starts with shopping, will require time
and endurance.

Boots

SELECTING BOOTS
Boots are your scaffolding. Do not skimp. Buy them from experts
who are informed, patient, and likely to be pleasant about returns.

With three months to go, my journey starts with Ed, the proprietor of a
local "outdoor motion" store. "Boots," he says, "need to fit more than feet.
They need to fit the person."

Like a physician taking a medical history, Ed asks about my hiking
and travel plans, while palpating the battered, hybrid boots that I use for
day hikes and have brought with me for his inspection. His expression is
grave.

"These won't do for the kind of walking you have in mind," he says,
bending a floppy sole in half. "They'll give you about as much support as
high-top sneakers. Let's see if we can do better." He begins pulling boxes
from the shelves.

We work for more than an hour before he rises from his boot-fitting
bench and suggests that I try another store with a wider selection. I'm
impressed with his sincerity and plan to return to purchase other gear. As
I leave, feeling dejected, Ed tries to reassure me. "Buying boots," he says,
"is serious business. Give it some time."

A few days later, in a mountaineering store an hour away in Burlington, Vermont, I'm staring at another wall of boxes, this time with Dave waiting to assist me. Eventually, I find a pair of boots that's almost right. After almost two hours, I'm tired and fading. I decide to take them home.

I walk around the house in my new, almost-right boots for a few days before admitting to myself that they won't do. I phone Dave, who analyzes my problem and places a special order for identical boots in a wider width.

A week later I'm back in the boot section with Dave assessing my feet, comparing the "not-quites" with the "special-orders." No need for make-do's or rationalizations this time. The wider boots fit my feet and my aspirations.

How do I know they're the right ones? Well, they feel right. A half-size larger than my street shoes, they are the lightest boots I can find with the support and protection I need. And they pass all the tests I learned from Ed. (See Tip 2.1.)

Dave concurs that these are the boots for me. Rather than being merely water resistant, they have a breathable (GORE TEX®), waterproof lining, a feature I will soon come to appreciate. They are also leather and have seams less likely to leak and tear than those on fabric boots. Dave assures me that leather breathes as well as fabric, once fabric has been waterproofed and its pores clogged with mud. Best of all, my boots look sensible, determined, and ready to trek for miles.

TIP : 2.1 ED'S TESTS FOR PROPER FIT

· Try on your boots while wearing the socks, sock liners, and innersoles you plan to use on your ramble. (Learn more from Tips 2.2 and 2.3.)

· Put on your boots. With the boots unlaced, push your toes into the front of each boot. If you can slip a finger into the space behind each heel, the boots are long enough.

· With toes pointed upward, tap the heel of each boot against the floor to bring your heel back into the heel cup. Now, lace your boots snugly, but not so tightly that circulation is restricted. Can you wiggle your toes? Does your arch feel comfortable?

- Walk down the incline the store should provide. If your toes feel cramped or if they jam against the front of the boot, try a larger size.
- Your heel shouldn't lift up more than a half-inch while you're breaking in your boots; it should lift even less once they are walking-ready.

Breaking in Boots

It seems that the longer it takes to break in new boots, the longer they are likely to last—but the longer I'm likely to worry about whether they're the right ones for me.

Nothing is quite as comforting as the certainty that new boots really fit. The fact that they do becomes clear to me on a boot break-in walk rather suddenly. It is the moment when I stop worrying about pinches and pressure points, ignore the stiff weights laced to my feet, and begin thinking about what to make for dinner.

Breaking in today's rather forgiving boots is not the blistering torture it once was. I begin by walking around the house late in the day when my feet are likely to be swollen. If the boots feel painful or bothersome, I return them. If I gradually forget I'm wearing them, chances are they will be fine.

I progress to fair-weather walking in the yard and some short walks around the block. Then I begin adding distance. Walking several miles gives discomfort a chance to nip at my heels. All this time, I continue "training" the tongue of the boots to lie straight beneath the laces.

I put miles on my boots by wearing them on daily walks. In this way I get to know their idiosyncrasies while I'm still in home territory. One pair, for example, made the ball of my foot numb for the first quarter of a mile. Then they were fine. I walked hundreds of happy miles in those boots.

After their distance trials, I treat my new footwear to their first waterproof coating and head out for a rainy day test. If they pass, we're ready to go. If not, I treat them again with an additional coat of waterproofing.

TIP : 2.2 FINE TUNING

· If your boots feel tight, try loosening the laces, or wear a lighter pair of socks. Boots feel tighter when socks are new or just washed.

· If a tight spot remains after your breaking-in period, a shoe repair shop with a mechanical boot stretcher might help. But for boots with breathable, waterproof linings, stretching may not be possible.

· If you prefer more cushioning, replace your boot's original innersoles with ones that are more to your liking. (See Tip 2.3.)

TIP : 2.3 CUSHIONING YOUR SOLE

· Feel free to remove and replace the innersoles that come with your boots.

· Choose innersoles you prefer or ones your salesperson recommends.

· You can purchase innersoles in shoe repair shops, pharmacies, and wherever boots are sold.

· Innersoles are variously constructed to provide cushioning and to support arches and heels.

· At the end of a day of walking, remove your innersoles for airing.

TIP : 2.4 WALK ABOUT

· To test your new boots, walk several miles in them—off road, if possible.

· Hilly, uneven ground is especially good.

· If you drive to the start of your walk, wear regular shoes for driving.

· Carry each boot in its own plastic bag.

· At the end of your outing, your car will be cleaner if your wet, muddy—perhaps smelly—boots ride home in those bags.

· Wipe or rinse mud and soil off your boots before putting them away.

· Do not store boots in plastic bags. They like to breathe.

Caring for Boots

It seems like there is more advice on the care and feeding of both leather and fabric boots, than on child rearing and dog training combined.

Be sure to ask the folks where you buy your boots how to care for them. Purchase with your boots all the lotions and waxes you'll need to keep them happy. While you're shopping, buy an extra pair of boot laces, and check out the store's selection of innersoles, socks, and sock liners.

Tip : 2.5 Little Things That Keep Boots Happy

- Clean and condition your leather boots occasionally with saddle soap or another moisturizing treatment recommended for boots.
- Waterproof your boots with a product formulated for leather or the type of fabric they're made of.
- Remove and dry your innersoles at the end of a day of walking. Turn your boots over and shake them to remove blister-causing pebbles and sand.
- Dry boots away from direct heat. Mine prefer afternoon sunshine.
- Store your boots in a dry place.

Socks

There are more good socks than there will ever be feet to wear them.

Just beyond the boot center, you spy a display of socks hanging from plastic hooks like ornaments on a Christmas tree. These are serious socks, padded in specific places for technical reasons, constructed for hikers, trekkers, and light trekkers. But which are you? How do you know if your heel and arch need more cushioning than your toes?

Do not despair. Socks are easier to buy than boots. Just ask your salesperson to suggest a pair to complement your boots.

When I ask Dave, he suggests the same socks I used for trying on my boots. I buy a pair of these. I also buy another, thicker, pair that he says will continue to cushion my feet as the socks wear.

Even a confirmed worrier need not be concerned about modern socks designed for recreational use because virtually all of them are technical wonders. They are all good. And they all work. It's just that some will work better for you than others. Walking in them as you break in your boots and limber up for a holiday on foot will reveal which ones are best for you.

Over many miles, I've walked in more than a dozen different kinds of socks and been pleased with all of them. My current favorites, a merino wool blend, are sturdy as well as comfy. And they don't shrink when I wash them or throw them into a dryer at the end of a rainy day walk, a real plus for someone who prefers dry socks in the morning.

Unfortunately, many of the socks you'll want to try on are packaged in a diabolical way that makes them virtually inseparable. So you may have to buy a pair before you test them. Since they are relatively inexpensive and useful for many activities, sock shopping is not much of a risk.

But wait. You also need a pair of lightweight, quick-drying, sock liners to wear under your new, heavier outer socks. Thin liners reduce friction and wick moisture away from working feet. They are your first defense against blisters. Even when you can't wash your outer socks, you will always have time to rinse and dry your light, inner ones. My favorites are ones that feel soft and fleecy, have some elasticity, dry quickly, and don't add much bulk or warmth.

Okay. You've done it. Boots, socks, liners, and maybe a set of innersoles. Time to put them all together to enjoy a walk on the mild side.

Tip : 2.6 Sock Sense

- Try out a few. And don't worry. They're probably all good choices. Just choose the ones you like.

- Wear two socks with your boots: a thin liner for wicking moisture and preventing blisters and a heavier, outer pair for comfort and cushioning.

- Every evening, wash your liners. Turn your heavy socks inside-out to air.

- Wash your outer socks when they will have time to dry or when a dryer is available. I wear mine about four days before washing them.

- Wear gaiters (see below) to protect socks from dirt, water, and abrasion.

Gaiters

Gaiters are the best friends boots and socks have.

Gaiters are removable, fabric sleeves with elastic ends that fit over the tops of boots and around the lower leg. They are essential. They never add weight to my pack because I wear them every day. Rain or shine, I zip them over my shoes, snapping the top and bottom of each into place. Mine are only mini-gaiters, about six inches high, without a waterproof coating, but they perform well in all kinds of weather.

Their lower edge has a hook that fastens onto boot laces. Their top edge rests on my leg when I wear shorts, or over my hiking pants when it's cool enough for me to put on long pants. My rain gear fits easily over them.

Gaiters can be a bit warm, but I ignore this because of the services they provide for me—and my feet.

⚜ J o u r n a l

Safe Socks

This has been a classic day in the Cotswolds. We've walked by thatch-covered cottages in storybook villages. The day has been warm and bright, the trails dry. I'm walking in shorts and a tee shirt, the first time I've been warm enough to indulge in such undressing.

Over Mike's objections, and feeling frisky, I leave my gaiters in my pack. A bad idea. I stop twice before lunch to remove sand and stones from my boots. My socks, which are supposed to go another two days before washing, are filthy, leaving no doubt that whenever I kick up my heels, I kick up a lot of dirt with them.

While Mike goes off, wearing his gaiters, to explore a side trail, I settle onto a rock to remove and shake out my socks and liners again. I empty pebbles from my boots and wipe off my innersoles. Then I dig out my gaiters and zip them on.

I believe Mike notices the change. But having won his point, he refrains from declaring victory as we head off for an afternoon of pebble-free walking. 🦡

Packs

Our loads seem lighter when, like us, the packs we carry are well adjusted.

As I stare at a wall hung with packs of all sizes and functions, I realize that I've never owned a real pack, one with a frame and with straps for adjusting everything except my attitude, which seems to be growing more sullen by the moment. Whatever I'm getting myself into looks like more than I want to carry.

Enter Jack, pack man of the mountain sports store in which I'm hyperventilating. Jack knows an overwhelmed soft adventurer when he sees one. In an attempt to reassure me, he says that he's just readied an entire expedition to climb Denali in Alaska.

Great. But can he outfit a what-if walker heading off to England?

He's not sure. He's adventurous, however, and would like to try. We approach the wall together.

FUNCTION

Our first decision is an easy one. For a countryside walk without luggage service, I will need more than a rucksack or day pack, but—thank goodness—less than an expedition model. Jack suggests a pack with an internal frame that is supposed to transfer weight from my back and weak shoulders onto my comparatively stronger hips. With its wide hip belt and padded back, it should feel comfortable as I balance on shaky legs and wobbly feet over uneven ground. The padding, which Jack says will warm my back on chilly days, will probably make me sweat on warm ones—the first of many tradeoffs.

SIZE

Jack is asking me how much I expect to carry. While I'm thinking about which items a woman who fills a canvas boat bag just to do her daily errands will need for a two-week walk, Jack turns to Mike, who is making pack decisions of his own. They are soon deep into a discussion of loads and cubic inches. Eventually, they return to something I understand: pounds. How many pounds can I comfortably carry? Time to find out.

On goes a pack. Into it Jack dumps coils of climbing rope. We get to about twenty pounds, and I'm still standing. At thirty, I'm sagging. He removes some rope. We decide my limit is twenty-five pounds for a walk I'm planning to enjoy. I'm a 3,000-5,000 cubic inches kind of girl.

STYLE AND COLOR

Having had lots of experience loading and unloading grocery bags, I opt for a top-loading pack. It has a narrow profile—no mesh water bottle holders or pockets sticking out from its sides to snag on branches and barbed wire or hinder my ability to negotiate narrow stiles and kissing gates. It also has two long, external tube-shaped pockets down the back where I'll be able to stow my rain gear and a water bottle. And it has a handy, zippered top compartment where I can stow my purse and lunch.

I prefer a bright color, but settle for aqua. Another tradeoff. (I'll have to accessorize.)

FIT

The fourth set of decisions is Jack's. My aqua pack has to be fitted to my body—shoulders, hips, and the length of my back. It's easier getting fitted for a wedding gown.

Jack selects one pack, then another. He replaces shoulder units and hip belts. He loosens this and tightens that, asking how this feels and if that rubs. I want to say "fine" to please him and because we're both getting tired. But my back and my vacation are at risk, so I force myself to concentrate and to try to be honest.

"Not good." "Not bad." "Okay." And, finally, with twenty pounds of climbing rope reinstalled, "Why, I hardly know it's there."

When I turn to the mirror to admire my outerwear, an outdoors-woman stares back at me. She looks absolutely beautiful!

OPERATION

Donning my new pack is like stepping onto a sailboat. Before getting underway, lines have to be rigged, hauled, and trimmed. Mike, who is prancing about the store, treating his own pack like an old friend, assures me that the black, nylon spaghetti hanging off mine has a purpose that will soon become clear. With Jack's coaching, I start adjusting things. I take in a compression strap, loosen a shoulder buckle, tighten a chest strap, and cinch in my hip belt so tightly that I have to loosen it, remove my pack, visit the bathroom, and start again.

At last I'm launched, trimmed, and on course, beating securely to windward. The pack is mine. A new friend, wrapped around me like a big, warm hug.

ACCESSORIES

A smart woman with a hefty line of credit once told me that she never buys a dress without the shoes, belt, purse, stockings, and scarf to go with it. I don't usually shop this way, which is why I'm never quite "put together." But I make an exception for my pack, which I accessorize as soon as I adopt it and before I leave the store.

First, I buy a small, external pouch, which will be worn on my left side below my waist, attached to two of the straps that still dangle down my chest. In it, I will place things I want to have at-the-ready: camera, lip balm, hand wipes, tissues, coins, candy, and an energy bar.

Next, I select a red nylon stuff sack for my sandals and a yellow one for my fleece jacket. I buy a metallic pink carabiner for clipping on my hats when they're not in use, along with a color-coordinated bright pink strap—as if I really need another strap—in case I want to secure something to the outside of my pack.

My final purchase is less fashionable, but more essential, than my pretty pink accessories. I buy a rainproof pack cover in case my pack's water-resistant material cannot hold up to the wallop of a British downpour.

Tip : 2.8 Pack Principles

> · Choose a pack that has room for all your belongings and is
>   easy to load.
> · It is better that a pack be too big and a little empty than too
>   small and always stuffed.
> · Comfort is critical, meaning correctly fitted and appropri-
>   ately sized.

Walker's Choice
Day Pack (Rucksack) or Backpack (Hiking/Trekking Pack)?

A few years ago, when I did some day hiking on a tour in New Zealand, I took along a small day pack, or rucksack. I vowed I would never use one again. Hanging that twelve pound rucksack on my weary shoulders was more uncomfortable than a twenty-three pound pack carried with the help of an internal frame and hip belt. Apparently, eight to ten pounds is my personal rucksack limit. Anything heavier, and I reach for a more substantial pack. A larger pack may not look as "cool" as a day pack, but at the end of an active day, my shoulders are a lot happier if I carry one.

I used my day pack again on another tour that included five days in the Peruvian jungle. This time a rucksack was the right choice. Our group of five traveled by boat most of the time. Our walks were short, our packs light. We didn't carry extra layers (it was ninety degrees) or rain gear (we wore it or just got wet). Even my light pack felt like too much to carry in the heat.

Tour companies usually recommend that their clients carry day packs. For New Zealand, the company's advice was poor. For Peru, however, it was just right. What's a traveler to do?

Tip : 2.9 Quick Test—Which Pack for Me?

> · Try to imagine what you'll be carrying each day on your
>   walk. Gather it up, and put it into your day pack. Is there
>   enough room for all your belongings and a little extra space
>   for something you might acquire along the way?
> · If everything fits, take your day pack out for a nice, long
>   walk. How do your shoulders feel?

- A day or so later, add some extra weight, just in case you forgot something the first time (full water bottle? camera? lunch? notebook? jacket?). Then take another walk. Still okay? Great. You're a "day packer."
- Not great? Time to shop for a backpack with a padded hip belt and a frame (internal or external). Your new pack may look larger than is fashionable, but you won't care. There's something liberating about choosing what works.
- If you're traveling with a companion, one frame pack may suffice. One of you can carry this, and the other can wear a rucksack or waist pack. Two friends of ours walked across England this way. They are still happily married, but they tell me that it's best to decide in advance which of you will play the role of Sherpa.

TIP | 2.10 PACK FACTS

DAY PACKS, RUCKSACKS, AND BOOK BAGS

- are useful for carrying lighter loads
- are designed to place weight on the shoulders
- can be carried on-flight or folded to fit into checked luggage
- do not have a rigid internal or external frame
- have lightly padded shoulder straps, but generally no "harness" strap between them
- may have a waist strap but will not have a hip belt

BACKPACKS OR HIKING/TREKKING PACKS

- are designed to transfer weight to the hips
- are useful for larger or heavier loads and for weak shoulders like mine
- may be too large to take as a carry-on, but can be laid flat inside checked luggage
- have internal or external frames
- have well-padded shoulder straps connected with an adjustable "harness" strap
- have a sturdy, padded hip belt
- have external (and perhaps internal) compression straps

Note: The British may refer to all packs as "rucksacks."

Getting Familiar

My pack sits on a chair in the kitchen, collapsed and harmless. I release its compression straps, stuff an old blanket into its cavern, and watch it swell with purpose. Balancing it on the kitchen counter, I back into its shoulder straps, tighten what I think needs adjusting, and feel it press against me like intimate apparel. The moment has come for us to take a walk together.

♦ J o u r n a l

Pack Pal

Day One: Ten pounds on my back. Three miles of walking.
The pack's weight rests on my hips as promised. But my arms are numb. I can't seem to adjust the correct straps. This is not going to work. We're never going to be friends. I feel like I have a monkey clinging to my back.

One Week Later: Ten pounds. Four miles.
I ease my shoulder straps, tighten the special straps that reduce the distance between my pack and my back, and cinch my hip belt. No numb arms. I can even move my shoulders. I feel hopeful.

Two Weeks Later: Ten pounds. Five miles.
Usually I'm comfortable carrying my pack, but not on this walk. The pack has added about ten degrees to the ambient temperature. I'm heating up. I need to remove my jacket. First, however, I have to remove my pack. It's a hassle, but has to be done. The drill commences: loosen straps, remove pack, stow jacket, close pack, put on pack, cinch waist belt, adjust straps. Not as much hassle as I expected, but next time I'll wear less.

Later Still: Fifteen pounds. Three miles.
My pack and I receive a lot of attention. People stop to ask why I'm wearing it. I say only that I am training for a long hike. When they ask about the miles I expect to walk, I answer, "as many as I can in ten days." The real number, one hundred, is still too daunting to say out loud.
  They also want to know how many pounds I expect to carry. "Don't

---

know yet," I tell them. "I'm guessing about twenty." (I'm hoping no more than twenty.)

Drivers smile as they go by. Do they think I look odd? Do they think I look rugged? Rugged would be nice. It's something I've never looked before.

A Lot Later: Fifteen pounds. Eight miles.

My pack and I have finally accepted each other. It embraces me like a friend after a long journey. It's my extra arm for carrying things. Its weight, resting on my hips, seems to buoy me up, rather than drag me down. Along with my terrier, it's become my companion on walks. I talk to it—a little embarrassed when I do—about the adventures we'll share and the places we'll visit together. We've become a team. ※

TIP : 2.11 SLOW AND STEADY PACK TRAINING

- Getting into shape for walking with a pack is an exercise in common sense.
- Keep your pack light, and walk a few miles.
- When you add a little weight, reduce your miles. Then add the miles back as you strengthen and gain balance.
- Build fitness slowly. Walk with your pack two or three times a week if you can.
- If you can't train gradually (and Mike never does), no one is going to punish you. Your trip will still be wonderful. You may have a few early aches, but you'll have plenty of time to get into condition as you ramble in comfort across the countryside (assuming that you're carrying a sensible pack that's right for you).
- Be sure you feel secure and strong before adding dog walking to pack training. One unexpected tug from a squirrel hunter can set back your training while you wait for bruises to heal.
- Time and weather permitting, take a long walk with a full pack about a week before you leave. The purpose of this exercise is to reassure. After completing it, confidence will be yours.

TIP : 2.12 CARRYING A BACKPACK

- As Mother used to say, "Watch your posture." Shoulders back, tummy in. Stand tall and straight.

- If you must bend forward, bend from your hips, not from your waist. Imagine you're walking into the wind. (This may not require much imagination!)

- When climbing hills, remain as upright as possible, and let your legs do the work.

- When lifting a pack, protect your back.
  - Bend your knees whenever you lift or remove your pack.
  - Avoid bending sideways.
  - Avoid twisting.
  - Never swing a pack onto your back.

- When putting on your pack, ask someone to lift and support it while you back into it. If you're alone, place it about waist-high on a wall, or lean it against a rock or other convenient surface (taking care not to damage its fabric) before slipping your arms through its straps.

- When removing your pack, ask a friend to support it, or find a friendly wall, rock, or grassy bank, and slip it off against one of these.

- A pack is not a purse. Carry yours on both shoulders.

TIP : 2.13 LOADING A BACKPACK

- Put clothing and other items into stuff sacks or plastic bags (rolled to remove the air and secured with rubber bands). Sort items into categories (underwear, socks, etc.) to keep things organized within.

- Loosen all straps before loading.

- Pad sharp items with clothing, and place them where they won't poke into your back or damage fabric.

- Place water bottles where you or a friend can reach them without your having to remove your pack. Ditto for your camera, tissues, candy, change, and other items you'd like to keep handy under way.

- Place heavy things up high inside your pack and close to

your back. But take care not to make your pack so top heavy that you feel off-balance.

· Tighten and adjust all compression straps before putting on your pack. Adjust your hip belt, shoulder, and other "traveling" straps after your pack is on.

Walking Sticks (Poles)

Aside from Mike, my favorite traveling companion on a ramble is my walking stick. I love everything about it: how it feels, the balance and stability it provides, and the way it builds arm strength without the grimness of resistance training. It's like having the power and drive of an extra leg.

I walk with a single metal pole, which I use in an ambidextrous manner. I wipe it off and collapse it down to baton length at the end of the day as we approach our bed and breakfast. The next morning, as we depart, I telescope out its segments, and off we go.

This is not my only stick. I own several traditional, hand-carved wooden ones, which I use on walks at home. These include a beauty I unearthed in a Yorkshire village. Regrettably, my special sticks are heavier and harder to pack than today's collapsible technical marvels.

The one I rely on came in a set of two. Mike walks with its twin. Together the four of us have traveled over nine hundred miles. Our sticks march to the music we sing. They seem to know when we're tired. They support us when we're not certain we can support ourselves. And they remind us that, when there are hills to climb, it helps to have others to lean on.

TIP : 2.14 WALKING STICK WAYS

· Walking sticks are necessities. They make walking safer and easier.

· You only need one pole, but will appreciate using two if you have knee problems.

· Two sticks are especially helpful when your pack is heavy, your legs are tired, a trail is steep, or the ground is muddy.

- Modern telescoping poles are easy to pack and light to carry.
- Look for poles with internal springs. Springs act like shock absorbers.
- If you and your stick are out in the rain, both of you should dry off before turning in for the night.
- A stick's pointed end is great for traction, but dangerous for eyes and exposed shins. Take care.

Shopping
On-line, in Store, or by Catalog

Although I'm a dedicated catalog user, I prefer in-store shopping when I'm unsure of what I'm doing and sense that I'm in over my head.

For my first "gearing up" experience, I was fortunate to have Ed, Dave, and Jack as my guides. Had I been left alone to forage through catalogs or to shop on-line without knowing what to ask—overwhelmed by numerous decisions, inadequate information, and the complexity of merchandise returns—I might have given up before taking my first step!

My friend Susan is my opposite. She is a dedicated at-home shopper. If it isn't on-line, she isn't interested. She bought her first pair of boots on the Web, put them on, walked in them for two miles, and left for New Zealand. She's a "what-me-worry?" gal, who seems to get away with such things.

If I tried shopping like Susan, I'd either be unshod or limping around on a foot full of blisters.

It's your call: the kind of shopping that works for you is best for you.

TIP : 2.15 CLARIFYING QUESTIONS FOR SHOPPERS
- Is this your first walking adventure? Your first pair of boots? Your first pack?
- How much help do you think you'll need to gear up?
- Can you get enough assistance over the phone or on a website?

- Are there stores in your area that can help outfit you?
- How do you feel about taking time to shop in person?
- Do you prefer to shop from home?
- Have you shopped "long-distance" for technical gear before?
- How well do you handle sending things back?
- Do you have enough time to order and reorder before you leave?

Moving On

Now that we've geared up, it's time to get ourselves dressed and decide what we need to take and what we can leave at home. For this, we move on to Step Three.

Step 3

Getting Ready
Kit and Caboodle

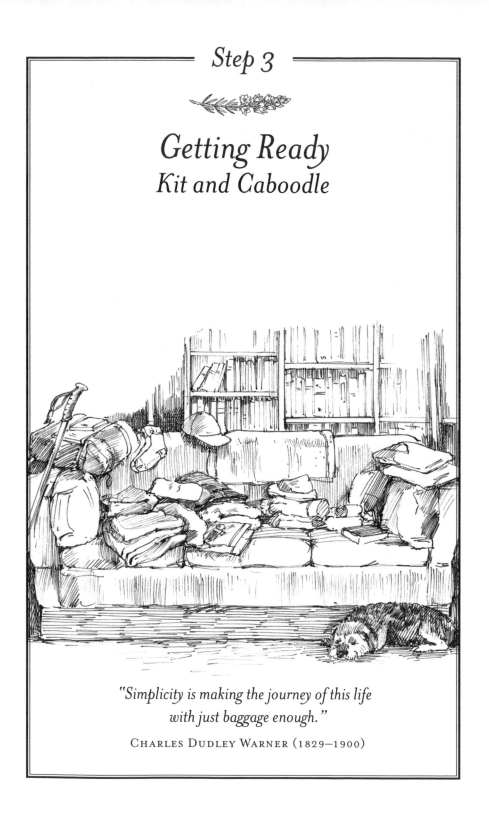

*"Simplicity is making the journey of this life
with just baggage enough."*

<small>CHARLES DUDLEY WARNER (1829–1900)</small>

Clothing

A Layered Life

Money and Travel Documents

Gadgets and Gizmos

Essential Incidentals
Water Containers
General Stuff
Optional Items We Usually Leave Behind
First Aid Kit
Toiletries
Et Cetera

Decision Time

Leftovers

Light and Lean
Mike's Short List
JoAnne's Even Shorter List

Moving Forward

Clothing

As questions go, "What should I wear on a countryside walk?"
creates a lot more anxiety than "What should I make for dinner?"

Bare Necessities

Four weeks to go, and I'm still writing lists. I've crossed off boots, socks, packs, and poles. This leaves clothing and "stuff." My plan is to gather everything together, spread it across our living room sofa, edit out redundancies, add items I've forgotten, and produce a final draft I can carry, one that Mike won't condemn as "more than one person will ever need." At least that's the plan. 🦟

LISTS FOR ALL REASONS

I thought I was in trouble when my girlfriend Tina sent me a copy of a backpacker's handbook filled with lists and illustrations of appealing gear that I have neither the pack space nor muscle power to carry. Happily, I won't be needing dehydrated food, climbing rope, or a camp stove on a countryside walk in the relative warmth of early fall.

Another helpful friend, recently back from a walk in Britain, handed me a list of the items she carried on her walk. I plan to sort through her suggestions and discuss them with Mike. Then I'll try to pare down my own list to approximate hers.

As I gather my gear, I am remembering the Sally Principle, and I'm leaving nothing (especially shopping) for the last minute. Named in honor of a friend who became frantic while packing for a trip to Vancouver the night before her departure, the Sally Principle holds that (1) the more thought we give to what we'll take on a trip, the less we're likely to take, (2) last-minute packing invites over-packing and is almost always stressful, and (3) stress is something travelers need to minimize.

JUST CALL ME "WICKIE"

I'm *stepping out* of, and leaving behind, most of what I own. I'm parting with familiar friends, like cotton tee shirts sporting rain forest insects and

"Save the Earth" messages. I'm leaving at home my jeans, sweatshirts (also with messages), and comfy cotton underwear. Cotton may be great in the tropics, but "up latitude" it doesn't retain body heat, dries very slowly, and gets mighty heavy when wet.

On a walk, creases are irrelevant, and wrinkles don't matter—only comfortable and practical matter. Dry and safe also matter. This is why "normal clothing" won't do.

So I'm setting off to hunt and gather in the commercial jungle—hoping I'll bag some smart-looking game suitable for covering a trekker. I'll be searching for hand-washable garments that breathe, wick moisture, dry fast (on a hanger or on me), won't melt in a dryer, and will fit into a pack.

I'm *stepping out* in backcountry fashion—into outdoorsy and casual, durable and sensible. I want performance wear that is light to carry and, regrettably, rather expensive. Fortunately, I don't expect to be buying very much of it, limited as I am by the volume and weight of my pack.

I'm starting on the outside and will be working inward until I reach the final and best layer, the perfect layer: my skin. It breathes, it wicks, it's washable, and, best of all, it fits. Remember—wrinkles don't matter.

TIP : 3.1 USED CLOTHING

· Before shopping for new things, review what you own.

· Unearth your forgotten, easy to wash-and-wear items.

· If your old favorites feel comfortable and you enjoy wearing them, take them. But only if you need them.

RAIN GEAR

Every once in awhile, rain gear may actually keep you dry.

· rain jacket
· rain pants
· waterproof pack cover
· light folding umbrella (optional)

Rain gear is not my favorite clothing. I don't like the reason I have to wear it, and I don't like the weight it adds to my pack when I'm not wearing it.

When the weather is wet and warm, I never know if I should put it on and sweat from the inside or leave it off and get drenched from the outside.

I really shouldn't complain. I carry great rain gear. It is waterproof with sealed seams, "breathable" (the only kind to walk in), lightweight, and brightly colored. It holds up well under a pack and is effective as a windbreaker. Unfurled and underway, however, it can be as noisy as a luffing jib.

I do not use a poncho to cover my pack or me. I find a poncho difficult to manage in heavy weather and a poor substitute for a raincoat or windbreaker. Ponchos are less comfortable and less effective than fitted rain gear combined with a pack cover. Pack covers are lightweight, waterproof (mostly), and easy to attach or remove in changing weather. I just wish they came in more exciting colors than boring blues, grim grays, and inoffensive greens.

I've considered adding an ultra-light, collapsible umbrella to use on warm, windless, showery days. Very tempting, especially when roaming village streets without my pack. So far, however, I've resisted.

As my rain gear and I walk together, we take care of each other. I wash away its mud to reduce fabric wear. It tries to keep me dry. But even after all our years traveling together, I can't say that we really like each other.

TIP : 3.2 IN CASE OF RAIN

- Keep handy your waterproof jacket and pants. They don't have to match.

- Carry these rolled up in separate plastic bags, so you can return them wet to your pack if the sun reappears.

- Put them on (at least your jacket and pack cover) when you feel the first drops of a shower. Assume that heavy rain will follow.

- Wear a cap with a brim under the hood of your rain jacket, especially if you wear eyeglasses. The brim will keep rain off your lenses, minimizing the need for frequent wiping, and will help you to see better from under your hood.

- Before leaving home, test your new rain gear in a rain storm or have someone spray you with a garden hose.

- Choose bright colors. They lift spirits on gray days and make motorists pay attention.
- Buy a jacket you'll also enjoy wearing on rainy day errands at home.

DRESSING UP

I'm about to tell you what I took with me on various walks, either worn on my body or carried in my pack. This confession is as personal as revealing my age (mature), weight (a bit too much), or income (not a chance). It's a struggle for me to be honest about packing because I'd rather cast myself as an adventurer, as a pro who travels light, rather than as the "what-if" person I am, inclined to pack more than I can comfortably carry.

Before you take my advice to heart and put the clothing I suggest on your back or into your pack, please note that my lists of what to take on a countryside walk are simply one woman's choices. Only you know what's best for you.

TIP : 3.3 SUITABLE CLOTHING: A DISCLAIMER

- Lists of what to pack are suggestions, not commandments.
- Edit my lists to reflect what suits you and makes you happy.
- Select comfortable clothing that fits well and that you'll enjoy wearing (and washing in a sink) over several days.
- Color is important. It cheers and invigorates.
- Cross off your list (and mine) everything you can leave behind. This exercise will make you stronger.

I have annotated my own lists of favorite things with comments (and a few excuses). My lists are followed by two others that are pared down for walkers more capable than I of traveling light. All three lists are based on the assumptions in Tip 3.4.

3.4 LET US ASSUME THAT...

- You will be carrying all of your own things. If you're using a luggage service or are on a tour that transports your luggage, you'll be able to take a number of extra items. I have suggested some of these extras at the end of my own, more Spartan, lists. (See "Leftovers.")

- You will not want to take time to leave the footpath to tramp several miles into town and back to purchase something you could have easily carried with you and might not be able to unearth in a small village (such as film, batteries, or boot laces).

- You will be walking with a friend with whom you can share the load. One of you, for example, can carry the medical kit, while the other carries the lunches. In the interest of full disclosure, I have listed in italics the items that Mike carried for both of us.

- Neither of you will carry more than twenty-five pounds, including water, lunch, and souvenirs.

- You will be walking in one set of clothes, but will carry a second set to wear to dinner while your walking wardrobe is airing or drying.

- Your clothes are capable of drying overnight in a chilly room and can also tumble in a hot dryer without melting.

- Your clothing is sturdy and easy to pack. You have walked in it at home with your pack on, and feel confident that it will last for the duration of your ramble without chafing or disintegrating.

A QUESTION OF AGE

I am fortunate. At this moment, I'm too old for tampons and too young for incontinence pads. This leaves more room in my pack for other things. But my age—which I share with Mike—makes its own demands. I need a hard case to protect a second pair of eyeglasses should my trifocals shatter. I need something warm to sleep in and clothes that dry quickly after an attack from a rogue hot flash. Mike needs a watch with a large face, and he needs pants with a built-in fly for ever more frequent stops along the way. We both prefer wearing pants with built-in belts or elastic waist-bands that adjust to changes in our figures as we eat, drink, and exercise along the way.

A Layered Life

OUTERWEAR
- fleece gloves and ski hat for cool weather
- sweatband
- baseball hat and/or sun protective hat that won't blow away
- fleece zip sweater-jacket
- ultra-light wind shirt
- fleece vest (optional)

Weather dictates where in my pack I place my outerwear. In cold temperatures my fleece jacket, hat, and gloves are near the top. On pleasant days I stow them at the bottom and keep my wind shirt handy.

I store clothing and gear in colorful, nylon "stuff sacks" or in plastic bags, which I roll (to remove the air) and secure with rubber bands. This makes things easy to organize and find—rather like having dresser drawers inside my pack. It's especially important to store rain gear and pack covers in plastic bags, because once the rain stops (which it will), you will be putting these things away wet (and often muddy).

I clip my hats and a sweatband on a pretty pink carabiner, which I attach to the outside of my pack. As I warm up or cool down and need to change head coverings, Mike removes my chapeau of choice from the collection and hands it to me. All my hats are brightly colored, so Mike can locate me if I go astray. Bright colors also look good in rainy day photos.

TIP : 3.5 HANDY PLASTIC BAGS
- Have on hand an assortment of bags. You'll need a selection of sizes.
- At home, before placing your clothes inside, spray a little scent on a paper towel and wipe the inside of the bag. Let dry. Enjoy "sachet on foot."

- With clothing inside, roll each bag to remove the air. Put a rubber band around the rolled bag to keep it compressed.
- Use bags to organize your clothing (underwear, socks, sleepwear).
- A large item (slacks, shirt) may require a bag of its own.
- Bags with "zippers" have sharp edges that can fray material. They are also difficult to fold. Although I rarely use them for clothing, Mike prefers them. They are, however, my first choice to protect and store travel documents.
- Reuse your nylon stuff sacks and plastic bags with abandon. They almost never require cleaning.
- Take along several extra bags (and rubber bands) for purchases, laundry, and to use when sitting on damp ground during lunch breaks.

PANTS

- one pair of walking shorts
- one pair of comfortable hiking pants
- another pair of hiking pants for evenings or back up

Everything I pack is made from synthetic fabric or is a cotton blend, quick-drying and light. I never wear cotton jeans, which are heavy, tend to be too tight for trekking, are downright uncomfortable when wet, and take forever to dry. All my trousers have pockets, and they are roomy enough to fit over long underwear bottoms if the weather gets chilly, and snug enough to fit under rain pants.

Many folks these days prefer tights, and these (as long as they are reasonably modest) also work well. I have noticed that some women have taken to wearing skirts or shorts with leg coverings beneath them. But I remain a plain pants/shorts gal myself.

Whatever pants you select, walk in them at home to make sure that nothing chafes and that you're comfortable wearing them with your pack. *Note: Pockets that end up beneath your hip belt will be inconvenient to access.*

Shirts
- two short sleeve tee shirts
- two long sleeve, lightweight travel shirts with pockets and with sleeves that can be rolled up, or one travel shirt and one long sleeve tee shirt
- one medium-weight, fleece, quarter-zip turtleneck

I like long sleeve shirts with pockets. They are versatile, with sleeves I can roll up or down for sun protection and for warmth or cooling as conditions change. I wear them over lightweight underwear or a quick-dry tee shirt. For climate control, I can turn up a collar or open some buttons. Synthetic fabrics that breathe keep me mostly dry, except under my pack where I am usually damp.

Lightweight tee shirts, made from today's miracle fabrics, are the perfect first layer. I wear one every day, either by itself or under a long sleeve shirt. For comfort and hygiene, I never wear a long sleeve shirt without a tee shirt under it. Most evenings, I wash out the tee I walked in and air out my outer shirt. Then I put on a clean tee and my spare long sleeve shirt, and head out for a hearty meal.

Usually, I get one or two days of wear out of a tee and about five out of a shirt before I need to wash them. If we are lucky enough to find ourselves at a B & B with laundry services, everything we've worn goes into a washer.

Underwear
- three underpants
- two bras
- one long sleeve, lightweight, quarter-zip turtleneck
- one pair of lightweight long johns (bottoms)

All the things that touch my body must wick, breathe, and fit. Some of today's synthetic fabrics retain odors more than others, so it pays to test (and wash) new intimate apparel before packing it.

I use the quarter-zip turtleneck to sleep in. When it's chilly indoors—and it often is—I sleep in my underwear bottoms as well. Occasionally,

I may wear my sleepwear under my pants and shirt for walking in cold weather.

Bras are my nemesis. Even the "wickiest" of them have some elastic in their construction. Long after everything else on me dries, a soggy, cold, elastic ring clings to my ribs like a boa constrictor. If I don't remove that wet layer soon after arriving at a B & B, I get mighty chilly and have a hard time warming up.

Although some women prefer a sports bra, almost any comfortable, well-constructed bra is fine for walking. Whatever style you purchase, make certain its straps and hooks (if there are any) won't irritate your skin when you're wearing a pack.

Footwear

- hiking boots with innersoles (extra innersoles optional)
- a set of gaiters
- three pairs of sock liners and three pairs of hiking socks
- shoes or sandals to wear in the evening while your boots are resting and drying
- socks that fit these evening shoes if your hiking socks are too heavy
- waterproof, nylon sock covers if your evening shoes are sandals
- an extra set of laces for your boots
- one pair of fleece socks

  Note: For suggestions and opinions about boots, socks, sock liners, and innersoles, please see Step Two.

What to carry for your second pair of shoes is a big decision. I have carried light sneakers and done well with them. But I also like rubber sandals with expandable straps. When it's warm, I wear them without socks. When it's cool, I put them on over a clean pair of hiking socks and adjust their velcro straps. They fit easily into my pack, weigh very little, and if they get wet, they dry quickly.

On rainy evenings, when I don't want to get my socks wet walking to dinner in sandals, I slip on a pair of soft, breathable, waterproof sock covers, which I discovered in a recreational clothing store. They fit comfortably over my socks and into my sandals and dry overnight for easy repacking.

I keep my sandals, socks, and waterproof sock covers in the same stuff sack in my pack.

For me fleece socks are an "essential." During the day I fold them in half and place one sock under each pack strap, just over my collar bone. Nothing makes carrying a backpack as comfortable as a pair of fleece socks padding its straps. And at night they keep my feet warm when I amble off to the loo.

ACCESSORIES

- colorful bandanna or scarf
- selection of earrings
- barrettes and/or hair ties if you have long locks
- wristwatch with a new battery installed shortly before leaving home

After a day on the footpath, it gives me pleasure to tie on a colorful scarf and add a fetching pair of earrings. These little props freshen my spirits and make me feel dolled up and ready to paint the town—even when I'm dressed in the same outfit I've been wearing for weeks. A bandanna is also useful during the day as a headband or as a mop for a wet brow.

Money and Travel Documents

- Local currency (bills and coins). Unfortunately, coins are heavy.
- Traveler's checks in local currency (pounds sterling for Great Britain). Most B & Bs do not accept credit cards.
- Passport. Make three photocopies of the inside cover (the page with your photo). Leave one copy at home with a friend. Carry a second, or give it to a traveling companion to carry for you. If possible, hide, lock, and leave a third in your luggage or in the hotel safe at your base camp hotel. (Read about base camp alternatives in Step Four.)
- Two extra passport photos in case you lose your passport and need to get a new one quickly. These, too, can be left behind at your base camp hotel.
- Credit/debit/ATM cards. Make two copies of each card. Remove your name from the copies. Leave one copy at home with a friend. Give the

other to a trustworthy traveling companion. Be sure to write on the copies the phone numbers to call if the cards are lost or stolen.

- Driver's license (if needed). Make two copies. If you can, place one copy in your locked base camp hotel luggage or a hotel safe. Give the other to a traveling companion.
- Trip cancellation insurance. If you purchase this, do so as soon as possible after purchasing your tickets. Take a copy of the policy with you.
- Plastic bags or other waterproof containers for carrying money and documents. Zipper-style bags work well for this.
- Security neck or shoulder pouch for important papers when you're in transit—not necessary (yet) while walking in the British countryside.

If you're walking through, or staying in, cities and need cash, ATM cards and dollar denomination traveler's checks will work just fine. But if you're in the "outback"—walking in the countryside, where ATM machines are as scarce as modern plumbing—you'll need to carry local currency.

Although most pubs, restaurants, and stores will accept credit/debit cards, most B & Bs, and many guest houses and inns, will not. Nor will your hosts accept U.S. dollars or dollar denomination traveler's checks because local banks charge a fee for exchanging these. B & Bs accept personal checks from British walkers. But, when it comes to us colonials, they expect either British cash or pound sterling traveler's checks.

TIP : 3.6 MONEY MATTERS

- The British countryside largely functions as a cash economy.
- Carry local currency and, if possible, pound sterling (local currency) traveler's checks.
- If you can, buy some currency and your traveler's checks before leaving home. Unfortunately, traveler's checks in foreign denominations are becoming difficult to purchase at banks in the United States.

Gadgets and Gizmos

Having lots of little things is nice. Carrying too many of them is not.

CAMERA — OPTIONAL

┌─────────────────────────────── ❦ J o u r n a l ─┐

Say "Cheese"

The Yorkshire Dales are laid out before me. A rainbow of greens framed by gray stone walls. I want to capture their rich openness. I want to take the bucolic scene home with me to revisit from afar.

Even though scenery is not its forte, I remove my small camera from the pouch attached to the front of my pack. I ask Mike to be my foreground and to pose on a four-step stile a few feet away. "One, two, three," I say. On cue, he turns and looks at me. Click. The Dales are mine. 🦡

My old 35 mm camera with its collection of heavy lenses would have taken a better picture. But when I carry a pack, point and shoot is what I do.

Even though I settle for less to keep my load light, I manage to take home images of the countryside I love—sometimes as photos, but more often as memories that stay with me wherever I go.

TIP ⋮ 3.7 PHOTOS ON FOOT

- Go light. A point and shoot camera saves ankles and knees.

- Practice your art before it counts. If your camera is new, don't leave home without snapping and viewing a few photos first.

- Rainy day pictures require rainy day cameras. If yours isn't waterproof, don't use it in a downpour.

- If you're carrying a standard camera, estimate the amount of film you will need. Then add a few more rolls. Because film is heavy, carry rolls of 36 exposures to reduce weight.

- Go digital if you can. Instant gratification is intoxicating.

- Digital cameras are light, although batteries and battery chargers can be heavy. (Film, however, can be even heavier.)

- Take more memory cards than you think you'll need because you will need them, even if you're planning to edit your collection each evening.
- Use your camera to capture images of people and local details.
- Supplement your photos with postcards, which generally do a fine job reproducing scenery.
- Walking is a beautiful subject for photography, so snap with abandon.

BINOCULARS — OPTIONAL

Mike and I both enjoy getting up close and personal with nature. On walks at home our day packs are never without binoculars and a field guide or two. When we travel, and if someone else is moving our belongings from place to place, we also keep binoculars handy in our light day packs. On a countryside walk, however, when we carry our worldly possessions on our backs, binoculars rarely make the final cut.

There are moments, of course, when we miss them—such as when we'd like to identify a bird or verify a waymark on a distant fence before walking across a wet field to find out if it's marking our path. Most of the time, however, we're happy to leave our binoculars at home and carry less.

CELL PHONE — USEFUL

I prefer to leave my cell phone at home. I don't like carrying its added weight and the weight of a charger. (For more on chargers, see "Charge It" below.) It's an intrusion when I'm trying to be in the here-and-now, focusing on the present. I especially don't like being tethered to demands back home, while immersing myself in a new experience.

Still, on our next walk we expect to carry one, which we plan to purchase at our overseas destination to ensure its compatibility with the local system. (See Step Fourteen, Facts Afoot.) As the familiar red British phone boxes slowly disappear and as we grow older, the need to reconfirm reservations, change plans, summon assistance, or arrange for transportation to off-trail lodgings makes cell phones more appealing and justifies carrying a little extra weight.

TIP : 3.8 CELL PHONE SURVIVAL

- Turn your phone off when walking. Let the countryside absorb you.

- Turn your phone on only when you need to make a call.

- Instruct loved ones back home that you are away and un-available. Ask them to call only in an emergency that you can mitigate from a distance or must know about before returning.

- If you're on a tour, and your leader is carrying a phone, turn yours off, or leave it in your luggage.

- If you are walking with a friend who is carrying a mobile phone, consider leaving yours at home or at the bottom of your pack.

- A walk is a perfect time for breaking an addiction to checking in and staying connected.

- Plug yourself into a new place by focusing on the path you're traveling. Step into freedom, into being discon-nected, into being only where you are.

GLOBAL POSITIONING SYSTEM (GPS) DEVICES — USEFUL

The decision to resist a GPS unit is a no-brainer for me. I'm low-tech at home and lower tech when I travel. I follow waymarks with the enthusiasm of a kid on a treasure hunt. I enjoy the simplicity of rambling along well-trod footpaths armed only with a map, a compass, and a trail guide. And I enjoy the luxury of having Mike, my very own human GPS device, as my companion, leading the way through bog and fog.

But the world is changing, whether I'm ready or not.

On our walk along the Welsh border, I had three companions: Mike, Robin (a British friend), and Robin's GPS unit, affectionately named "Offie," in honor of "his" digital assistance along the Offa's Dyke Path.

We consulted Offie often. We looked to him for sound advice, which he always provided. We relied on the accuracy of his information. Each night before Robin tucked him into his charger, we asked Offie to review the data of our day: elevation scaled, distance traveled, and the route taken.

Offie was a champ. He never failed or complained. He didn't get blisters. He didn't get hungry or tired. He told us precisely where we were and pointed us in the right direction. He also saved us a lot of guesswork when the trail was obscure or when we had to locate our lodgings or make an unforeseen diversion.

This we know: The next time Mike and I lace up our hiking boots for a long walk, we'll put an "Offie" in Mike's pocket to show us the way. After his help on the Offa's Dyke Path, we can't imagine leaving home without him.

CHARGE IT

The problem with gadgets is the power required to operate them. It always adds weight. Cameras, GPS units, mobile phones, and electric shavers all depend on some configuration of batteries, which often depend on chargers and conversion plugs. Some of these devices have been combined into a single gadget or designed so that they can plug into one universal charger. Still, electronic conveniences weigh heavily on the walker.

Our solution is to divide and reduce. We carry two cameras, but only one charger that fits both of them. When Robin, our British friend, walks with us, we three carry three cameras, one mobile phone, and a GPS unit (no electric shavers). These require three separate chargers and a conversion plug. Clearly, we still have a way to go.

We want to go lighter. We are motivated to do better. We are aware that every gadget, and the power supply required to "charge it," draws down our personal energy reserves. But at present, all we can do is wait until technology catches up with the simplicity of walking.

GADGETS: TAKE THEM OR LEAVE THEM

The challenge of packing is to figure out ahead of time which possessions are essential to take along (that is, which ones we need in order to feel safe, comfortable, and happy) and then to leave many of these "essential" items, and everything else, behind.

Essential Incidentals

In addition to clothing, we also carry a fair amount of "stuff," which we divide between us. As you make your own list, the items below may bring things to mind that you, too, would like to take along—or leave behind. The items Mike carries for both of us are in italics.

WATER CONTAINERS

There seem to be as many ways to carry water as there are thirsty walkers.

• We carry one liter of water per person in containers that are safe and convenient to use.
• We rinse out our containers each evening.

I carry a refillable, hard plastic, liter-size bottle. It fits nicely into an external, zippered compartment in my pack. The bottle is easy to clean and refill. After drinking and before stowing, I place it into a plastic bread bag, which I fold over and secure with a rubber band. Water has never leaked into my pack. When I want a drink, I either remove my pack or ask someone to unzip the compartment and hand the bottle to me—which is not a problem because there is usually someone with me to ask.

A better arrangement (except for problems caused by water bottles that protrude and snag on things—see Step Two, "Packs") is to carry water bottles in the external side pockets found on many packs today. When you want to grab a drink, you simply reach around and help yourself. Two half-liter bottles (one per pocket) work well. So do store-bought bottles of spring water that you can refill or recycle at the end of the day. Just be sure that the bottles fit securely into your backpack pockets and that you thoroughly clean and air dry your containers each evening.

Another increasingly popular option is the hydration pack, which fits into a backpack. Some backpacks now have special compartments (some external) to accommodate one. A tube from the water reservoir allows a walker to take in water without stopping to open and drink from a bottle. The system is convenient and easy to use.

Some of the drawbacks of this method of hydration are: (a) the unit can take up precious room inside a pack; (b) it is not easy to share your extra water with a friend; (c) the interior of the hydration pack must be kept thoroughly clean; and (d) walkers who drink while walking forfeit a splendid excuse to pause, relax, and take in the scenery—which is what vacations are all about.

Note: Buy your water containers (bottles or hydration packs) from sports outlets that offer a variety of them. Consult with sales people who know which ones are safest and which ones will be best for you. Be sure to ask how to keep yours clean.

General Stuff
- very small flashlight
- eyeglasses—a pair and a spare
- sunglasses if eyeglasses to do not have UV protection
- safety pins, rubber bands, twist ties, and paper clips
- a few extra plastic bags of various sizes
- lightweight line (such as parachute cord) for drying clothes in bedrooms
- flat rubber sink stopper
- candy and energy bars that won't melt in the heat or run in the rain
- hand sanitizing liquid or individual hand wipes
- small packages of facial tissues
- panty liners
- whistle
- lock for luggage left in rooms —only used occasionally
- ear plugs
- elastic ankle brace and knee brace
- *sewing kit*
- *small pocketknife*
- *compass*
- *small roll of duct tape for rips and mishaps*
- *tiny alarm clock if your wristwatch doesn't have one*
- *super lightweight emergency rescue blanket*
- *guidebooks and maps*
- *GPS device*

We each carry one ankle and one knee brace made of elasticized material, hoping that both knees (or both ankles) won't desert either of us at the same time. Carrying these gives me confidence, and, I think, a little luck. So far, I haven't had to use either one. But should an ankle or knee suddenly need support, we won't have to hobble to the next town in search of some.

I keep a "piddle pack" handy in an outside pocket. It contains several tissues, a sandwich bag, and a few hand wipes. (More about answering calls of nature in Step Ten.)

Optional Items We Usually Leave Behind
• laundry powder—we wash our laundry with hand soap
• a towel and a small piece of soap for overnights in youth hostels
• washcloth—most British B & Bs don't provide these
• nylon net or shower sponge for applying shower gel
• *small pair of binoculars*
• *cell phone*
Note: *For walks in exotic, tropical destinations far from Britain, we add bug repellent, toilet paper, and water treatment tablets.*

If I carry a towel, it is light, absorbent, and small. A backpacking towel works well. I have used one to wring out laundry at B & Bs that ration towels and have folded one around my neck on wet days to keep out drips of rain. Towels are a must at youth hostels, which do not provide them.

Many B & Bs do not provide bar soap or shampoo. Instead, you'll find liquid hand soap, body wash, and shower gel. You will almost never find a washcloth (a.k.a. flannel). So, if you need one, you'd best take one with you from home—in a plastic bag, of course.

First Aid Kit
• *moleskin*
• *lamb's wool*
• *adhesive bandages*
• *scissors that can double as toenail clippers*
• *antiseptic ointment or cream*

- *alcohol wipes*
- *gauze patches and tape*
- *tweezers and a needle*—essential for removing small thorns and splinters
- *blister patches*

What you place in your kit will depend on your own needs. We try to keep ours light. This isn't easy for a contingency planner like me, who thinks about all the things that could go wrong. Since Mike usually thinks about things going right, he's the one who pares down our kit to its essentials.

The best way to treat abused feet is a topic of endless debate among walkers. (Read more about this in Step Nine.) Mike and I prefer to wrap individual "problem" toes with a few strands of lamb's wool preventatively, or as soon as we are aware of a minor irritation. The wool felts to itself and doesn't require tape. Moleskin helps to protect heels and other areas not easily wrapped with wool. So we carry this, too, and use it occasionally. We also carry blister patches filled with gel to cushion hot spots and full-fledged blisters that occur despite all our precautions and good intentions.

TOILETRIES (*indicates an item we share)
- toothpaste and toothbrush
- dental floss
- deodorant *
- shampoo *
- comb and brush
- powder to keep toes dry and happy *—we prefer pure cornstarch
- emery board and nail file *
- ear swabs
- lip balm with SPF protection
- moisturizing skin lotion with UV protection *
- sunblock—for additional UV protection (optional) *
- mouthwash strips—only in cool climates (optional)

Whether your personal list resembles ours or not, the challenge here is that toiletries need to fit into a small zippered case, which will go into its own plastic bag and into a pack, which you will carry. The objective is to keep it light.

To save space, every bottle in my pack is mini-sized. I pour all liquids into these small plastic containers, which I place into sandwich bags secured with rubber bands to prevent spills.

To save weight, I take one small tube of toothpaste and make it last. My skin lotion doubles as sunblock. My comb and brush are small enough to fit into my very small purse. I use whatever shampoo and soap B & Bs provide and save my own micro supply for "just in case."

We like to carry mouthwash strips, but only on walks in relatively cool, dry climates. We discovered in the Peruvian rain forest that they melt and congeal when heated or exposed to high humidity.

Et Cetera

- makeup—I go basic: cover stick, compact with mirror, and a lipstick
- jewelry—a wristwatch and several changes of inexpensive earrings
- purse—small enough to fit into a pack
- medicines and nutritional supplements
  - We take only what we really need
  - We count out our tablets ahead of time
  - Plastic bags or bottles keep things dry and fresh
  - Prescriptions can be carried in their original (small) containers
- business items—notebook, pens, addresses, postcard stamps
- home photos (to show to new friends)
- book—I gave up carrying this extra weight when I discovered that I usually fall asleep before I get around to reading. If I'm awake, I read one of the books provided by our B & B, a guidebook, or the travel brochures we collect along the way and which Mike is nice enough to carry. When our collection weighs enough for him to complain, we package it, and mail it home to ourselves on a slow boat. (More about mailing things home in Step Ten.)
- foreign language phrase book—when needed

Decision Time

I used to think that packing was a matter of deciding what to take. But, given the finite space of my pack, the effect of weight on aging knees, and Mike's voice mumbling, "When in doubt, leave it out," I have come to understand that packing is really about what can be left behind.

Leftovers
Things We Might Add if We Were Not Carrying Them Ourselves

These are the optional items I miss the most when I look into my pack each evening and wish they were there.
- novel—for nights when I'd rather not read a guidebook, brochure, or a book off the shelf of a B & B
- hair dryer and converter—happily, many B & Bs now provide hair dryers
- standard size hair brush and comb
- sneakers and socks
- one turtleneck
- one more long-sleeve synthetic-blend blouse
- flannel shirt
- fleece vest
- two pretty cotton tee shirts
- third pair of long pants
- nightgown
- bird and wildflower field guides
- more souvenirs
- our dog—who watches us pack, nests in our travel clothes, and promises to behave if only we'd take him with us on a long country walk

Light and Lean

I asked Mike to write down the clothing and incidentals he carries. He handed me the list below along with a disclaimer: "I'll be taking even less on our next walk."

"Sounds like a good idea to me," I reply with a smile, having watched him jettison enough stuff before our last walk to qualify him for the "Bare Bones Award."

"And," he adds, but shouldn't have, "my lighter pack will be off-limits to overflow from the person walking with me, who might do well to reduce the contents of her own pack." I stop smiling, grab his smug little list, and walk away.

Mike's Short List

Outerwear
- rain jacket and pants
- gaiters
- waterproof pack cover
- ski hat (in cool weather)
- large bandanna
- sun protective hat that won't blow away
- ultra-light wind-shirt pullover
- light fleece vest

Pants (cotton blend or synthetic)
- one pair of shorts
- one comfortable pair of hiking pants, which Mike wears every evening. In cool weather he wears these for walking as well. He doesn't carry a second pair of long pants for off-trail use. My pleas of "What if they rip? What if they need washing? What if they get wet?" don't register with someone who once got very wet and dirty walking the Appalachian Trail.

Tops (cotton blend or synthetic)
- two tee shirts—also used as underwear
- two long sleeve, lightweight shirts with roll-up sleeves

Underwear (cotton blend or synthetic)
• two underpants
• one long sleeve, lightweight, quarter-zip turtleneck (in cool weather)

Footwear
• hiking boots
• three pairs of sock liners
• three pairs of medium weight, wool-blend hiking socks
• ultra-light sneakers to wear in the evening
• extra set of laces for boots

Stuff
• water bottle
• small packages of facial tissues
• very small flashlight
• eyeglasses—a pair and a spare
• extra plastic bags of various sizes
• elastic ankle brace and knee brace
• luggage lock
• digital camera with battery charger, memory cards, and adapter
• matches packed in plastic, zipper-type sandwich bags
• small pocketknife
• toiletries—selected by a minimalist
• two or three disposable razors and a minute supply of shaving cream
• first aid kit
• sewing kit
• small roll of duct tape for rips and mishaps
• candy and energy bars
• compass
• trail guidebook and maps
• GPS unit (now carried)

Not Carried…Yet
• cell phone
• small pair of binoculars

JoAnne's Even Shorter List

JoAnne and her husband Bob have walked in Ireland, France, and England (several times). A few years ago, JoAnne carried a pack that exceeded my own twenty-five pound limit. She resolved, however, to cut back and reduce the load on her knees in order to increase the pleasure of her walks, and she has been successful.

Her current packing list is a pared-down remnant of her past life on the trail. With her permission I have reproduced it here to recognize her achievement and to inspire over-packers everywhere. Keep in mind that hers is the list of a woman who is rarely cold and who, therefore, requires fewer layers than chillier mortals. She also feels she does not need to be a what-if kind of gal while traveling in England.

Still, her list is an example to emulate. I want to thank her for demonstrating how much the rest of us can leave behind.

Clothing
- two bras
- two underpants
- two pairs of sock liners
- two pairs of hiking socks
- three shirts (one lightweight wool)
- two hiking pants (no shorts)
- silk long johns—top and bottom (also used for sleeping)
- hiking boots
- off-trail shoes
- rain jacket (no rain pants)
- hat with a full brim

Stuff
- two half-liter water bottles
- contact lens cleaner
- extra eye glasses
- small manicure set
- bare essentials toiletries kit: deodorant, soap, shampoo, toothbrush, toothpaste

- makeup—limited to sunscreen and lip balm with UV protection
- travel kit with medicines and vitamins
- lamb's wool and moleskin for sore toes
- small digital camera and accessories: extra memory cards, charger, adaptor, waterproof pack for camera
- mini-purse for money, documents, passport, comb and brush
- envelope for lodging information, addresses, stamps, brochures
- book

JoAnne notes that she organizes into categories the items she carries and packs her things in zipper-style plastic bags. In the spirit of full disclosure, she confesses that husband Bob carries the following items to lighten her load:

- first aid kit
- maps
- lunches
- drink mixes and energy bars

Overlooked
I recently asked JoAnne if there were something she'd like to add to her list for her next walk. Without hesitating, she replied, "There is. A washcloth! I don't think the Brits believe in them."

Moving Forward

Our lists completed, our purchases made, we move now to Step Four, to the nuts and bolts of travel, to planning our itinerary and arranging evening accommodations along the footpath.

Step 4

Logistical Logic
Planning a Ramble

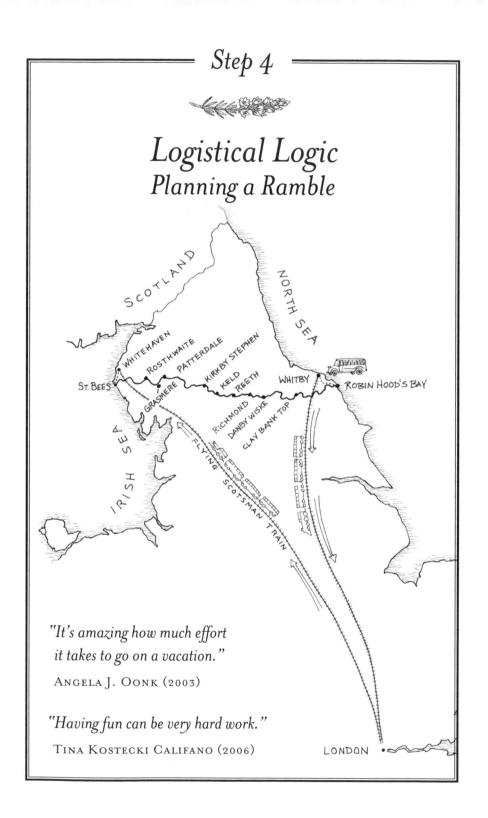

"It's amazing how much effort
it takes to go on a vacation."
Angela J. Oonk (2003)

"Having fun can be very hard work."
Tina Kostecki Califano (2006)

Ways to Go

In the Beginning
Option One: Package Plan
Option Two: Luggage Support
    Tɪᴘ 4.1: Luggage Service Limits
Option Three: Free and Easy

Base Camp Alternatives
    Tɪᴘ 4.2: "Just in Case" Packing
Base Camp at Point of Arrival
Base Camp at the Trail Head
Base Camp at the Trail's End

Beyond Base Camp
Principle One: Rate x Time = Distance
    Tɪᴘ 4.3: Setting the Pace
Principle Two: Information before Reservation
    Tɪᴘ 4.4: Locating Basic Information
    Tɪᴘ 4.5: Making Reservations
    Tɪᴘ 4.6: The Right Room for You
    One-of-a-Kind B & B—Dales Way
Principle Three: Rest Stops Matter
    Full Day at Leisure—Coast to Coast Walk
    Jᴏᴜʀɴᴀʟ: Losing It
    Full Day to Explore—Offa's Dyke Path
    Tɪᴘ 4.7: Ideas for a Getaway Day
Principle Four: Overseas Connections
    Tɪᴘ 4.8: Grandma Doesn't Have a Website
Principle Five: Confirming Reservations
    Tɪᴘ 4.9: Confirmation Basics
    Best Made Plans Go Awry
Principle Six: Managing Public Transportation
    Tɪᴘ 4.10: Tickets and Schedules

Whew! That's Done

Ways to Go

We're almost ready, but first we'll need to plan our itinerary. Where should we spend the first few days after our arrival? Will we be able to leave our overseas luggage there? How many miles will we walk in how many days? And what about making lodging arrangements for our ramble?

The pages that follow suggest alternative strategies to ensure a smooth transition from home to footpath. After reviewing these options, we'll consider six basic principles for planning a walk and making overnight reservations.

Where, then, are we to stay, and how far shall we walk each day? Let's just say, "It all depends."

In the Beginning

OPTION ONE: PACKAGE PLAN
LOGISTICALLY LITE

If you've decided to travel with a group, your packaged tour has made arrangements for your arrival and accommodations. So, put your feet up and humor the rest of us while you read this brief section and skim the rest of the chapter about planning an independent ramble.

Perhaps someone from your tour will meet you at the airport and help with the transfer of your luggage. If not, you've probably received directions to the hotel where you'll be spending your first night, and you will proceed on your own to that destination. There you will meet your fellow walkers and your guide, who will impart practical advice and help you settle in.

The following morning, you'll place some items into a light day pack and leave your luggage behind, confident that your abandoned belongings will meet you in your next room. After a generous breakfast, you'll depart with your new friends on the first day of your ramble.

May the sun shine upon you and the wind be at your back.

Option Two: Luggage Support
Unburdening Yourself

If you've opted for a self-guided walk with a luggage service to transfer your things, your plans for the first few nights will be flexible and uncomplicated. The following schedule is one that might appeal:

- Arrival day: Walk about and relax. Overnight in city of arrival.
- Second day: Travel to start of trail. Contact luggage service upon arrival.
- Second night: Overnight in village at head of trail; pack your day pack.
- Third day: Set out on your adventure carrying your day pack. Leave the rest for the luggage service to transfer to your next inn, B & B, or hotel.

If you have more energy than I do, you might choose to compress your plans and try this schedule instead:

- Arrival day: Travel to start of trail. Contact luggage service; overnight in village at head of trail; pack your day pack.
- Second day: Set out on your adventure carrying your day pack. Leave the rest for the luggage service to transfer to your next inn, B & B, or hotel.

Your luggage should be waiting for you when you arrive.

TIP : 4.1 LUGGAGE SERVICE LIMITS

Luggage services vary. So find out if yours:

- Picks up luggage at B & Bs in the communities on your personal itinerary.
- Drops off luggage at individual B & Bs, rather than at a central drop-off point in a village.
- Covers luggage that will be left outdoors in the rain to wait for you.
- Charges by weight or by the number of bags. (You may want to consolidate into one large duffel.)

- Plans itineraries and makes reservations. (This extra service for an extra fee can save you time and effort.)

- Reserves accommodations at locations that suit the number of miles you wish to walk.

- Is more economical and convenient than arranging for luggage transfers with B & B hosts and local taxi services, which you can do when you reserve your room.

Option Three: Free and Easy
The Minimalist Approach

This option never crosses my mind. But in the spirit of "whatever makes you happy," let me mention how Paul and Emily from Vermont begin their walks.

These intrepid wanderers place everything they're taking with them into their backpacks and arrive at the airport wearing their hiking clothes. They each carry a rain jacket, a paperback book, and a small purse into which they put their money and documents, a comb, some mints, and a pen. No change of underwear, no neck pillow, and no containers for prescriptions. Free Spirits don't carry medications or nutritional supplements. They're strong and healthy.

They are not what-if travelers. They don't spend time thinking about and preparing for what might go wrong. Apparently, they don't need to. At airport check-in, their packs, with their belongings inside, are shrink-wrapped, or placed into a carton, and checked through. These packs miraculously reappear in the baggage claim area, undamaged and on time, when Paul and Emily do.

At the airport, they unwrap their packs, deposit their paperbacks, raincoats, and purses into several empty compartments, and march out of the airport looking like the ramblers they are.

They spend their first day traveling to the trail head where they check into the B & B they reserved ahead of time. After only one night of rest, energized by a full English breakfast, they set off down the path.

Base Camp Alternatives
Gradual Beginnings

For a great start, make your first hotel the "base camp" of your expedition. This method works well for a tenderfoot like me, who needs a safe place to leave extra "just in case" items she doesn't want to carry for a hundred miles on her back.

TIP : 4.2 "JUST IN CASE" PACKING

- On your overseas flight, dress in clothing you can walk in—just in case your luggage doesn't arrive on time or at all.

- Wear your hiking boots—just in case your luggage is lost. It's too difficult to break in new boots (assuming you can find a new pair that fits). Loosen or remove your boots in flight, and wiggle your toes. Keep socks clean by wearing in-flight slippers.

- Pack an on-flight bag—just in case your luggage has to catch up with you. Put the following items into it: a change of underwear, something to sleep in, and an extra pair of sock liners; toiletries, medications, and a first aid kit; your fleece jacket, a raincoat, your camera with its accessories, and other valuables, such as binoculars.

- Take with you all of your airplane necessities (neck pillow, book, slippers, ear plugs, eye shade, water bottle, snacks, etc.)—just in case conditions in "steerage" deteriorate to intolerable. (For more on enduring an overseas flight, see Step Six.)

- Keep secure all money and documents—just in case other travelers are not as nice as you are.

- Place everything else in a duffel bag (with wheels) to be checked through. This includes your backpack, walking stick, and clothing. If you are traveling with a companion, consider sharing one large duffel. One bag is easier to manage and to store at your base camp.

- Be sure that your checked bag has been correctly tagged for your destination.

The location of your base camp will depend on your plans for travel. The following examples illustrate alternatives that have worked well for us.

Base Camp at Point of Arrival

- First day and night: Check into lodgings in your city of arrival. Wander about town and explore your surroundings. Before turning in, lay out your walking gear and the contents of your pack. Place inside your duffel everything else, which you won't be taking on your walk, but will want to have on your flight home or for sightseeing, should you decide to cut short your walk. I like to have waiting a clean set of clothes, a pair of sneakers, and a guidebook. I also leave my on-flight bag and flight pillow. Think of sorting and repacking at base camp as your last chance to jettison unnecessary items and lighten your pack.
- Next morning: Lock and leave your duffel at the hotel. *(Note: Some hotels now charge a daily fee per bag for this storage service.)* Pack your backpack. Fill your water bottle. Pick up your walking stick. Dressed in walking clothes and wearing your pack, proudly head for the train or bus that will take you to the trail head. We usually buy our lunches before boarding.
- Second night: Overnight in the village at the head of the trail. Try to sleep despite your excitement.
- Third day: Time for *stepping out.*
- At the end of the trail: Return to base camp to spend a night (or several nights, if you're doing some sightseeing). Collect your duffel, and repack for your flight home.

Using the Point of Arrival Alternative in London

Dressed for walking, we depart from our London hotel on the second morning of our stay. We take the underground to Euston Station. Here we board the Flying Scotsman to Carlisle, en route to the remote village of St. Bees, located at the start of the Coast to Coast Walk, where we have reserved a room for the night.

We arrive at three in the afternoon in Whitehaven, a town five miles from St. Bees. There are no taxis in sight. Jet lagged and dazed, we are considering our options when a tiny car pulls up to collect a young woman, the only other passenger on the platform. She asks if we would like a lift to our trailhead at St. Bees. Our packs, she says, are a giveaway. Her mother, our driver, invites us to jam our gear into the car's mini-trunk and squeeze ourselves onto its skinny back seat. Before speeding home, she stops at the market to buy a chocolate cake and some cold drinks, which she passes back to us to balance on our knees. We arrive at her home just after four and are invited to tea, which, of course, includes the chocolate cake. We have made our first "C-to-C" friends.

After tea, our host, who knows our B & B proprietor and everyone else in town, drops us at Mrs. W's door, pauses for a brief chat, and zips off—with my walking stick still in her car. I retrieve it later on our way to dinner. This gives us a perfect opportunity to meet the rest of her family—and a perfect start to our journey.

BASE CAMP AT THE TRAIL HEAD

- First day: Travel from the airport with all your luggage to the start of your walk. Overnight in the village at the head of the trail.
- Second day: Enjoy a leisurely tour of the village, and take a stroll to limber up. Before turning down your duvet for the night, request a packed lunch if you think you will need one for your first day of walking. Some hardy souls begin walking on the morning of their second day. We don't. We like having a day to rest and walk about. I'm just too travel weary to generate enough enthusiasm to support a positive attitude.
- Third day: Pack your backpack. Leave your locked duffel at your base camp hotel. Enjoy a full breakfast. You're as ready as you'll ever be for *stepping out*.
- At the end of your ramble: Return to your base camp hotel, collect your things, spend the night, and repack for the plane. The next day, travel back to the airport to return home (unless you're extending your visit).

Using the Trail Head Alternative in Ilkley

Convenient transportation is not always available from the end of a path back to the B & B from which you set off. But when it is, this option works well. We have used it several times. The first was when we walked the

Dales Way. From London's Heathrow Airport, we traveled directly to Ilkley to spend two nights at a small hotel.

When we arrive, our host is mesmerized by the telly. We drag ourselves in with our luggage. Eventually, she refocuses her attention and tends to our check-in with red eyes and minimal interest until the screen recaptures her attention. "Just awful, isn't it?" she keeps repeating. We have arrived on the day of Princess Diana's funeral.

The topic of conversation everywhere—in the tea room, book shop, tourist center—is focused on this tragedy. Still, we manage to order some tea and creamy pastries and purchase a pocket-size book of British history. We also discover a small, map-style trail guide of the Dales Way at the tourist information center. It is as light as a hiking sock and clear enough for me to follow without losing my way. In a decade of trekking, I've never found a guide as useful or as practical as this one. (See "Trail Guides" in Step Eleven.)

On our rest day we walk two miles to Addingham, the mill town that Mike's ancestors called "home" before they were displaced by the Industrial Revolution. We take time to read some of his family history, preserved on the weathered gravestones, but we cannot review old church records. The church office is closed for the funeral.

At noon, when the pub opens, we sample a local brew and fill up on jacket (baked) potatoes topped with tuna salad and baked beans. After lunch, we follow a different footpath back to our hotel in Ilkley. Before turning in, we sort, cull, and repack for our Dales Way walk.

Base Camp at the Trail's End

• First day: Travel from the airport to the community where your walk will conclude. Relax and enjoy the day. Confirm the details of the itinerary you plan to follow to reach the head of the trail. Before turning in for the night, sort your belongings and repack your duffel. Leave behind everything that is not going with you on your walk.

• Second day: Give your locked duffel to the manager/owner of your inn or B & B, and travel to the start of the trail on public transportation. Walk about and see the village.

- Second evening: Turn in early. You're rested and ready to begin your walk.
- Third day: After breakfast you set off, walking stick in hand.
- At the end of your ramble: You arrive at your base camp lodgings where you collect your things, repack for the plane, and spend the night. The next day, travel back to the airport to return home (unless you're extending your visit).

Using the Trail's End Alternative in Bath

From London's Heathrow Airport, we take an express train to Paddington Station, buy our lunches, and catch the next train to Bath, where we spend the afternoon visiting that most Georgian of cities. We head first to the abbey, which marks the official southern end point of the Cotswold Way. We admire its elegance, stare at a man, covered in silver paint, performing just outside, and enjoy a spot of tea at the nearby Pump Room.

We've come to the abbey to snap a "before" photo in front of its carved doors, which, if all goes well, we hope to visit again in a little over a week. We picture ourselves marching down Bath's main shopping street, crossing its busy plaza, and returning to these massive doors to take another photo at the end of our walk. In that photo we'll be wearing our packs, as we bid farewell to the elegance of the Cotswold Way.

But first, we have to make our way to Chipping Campden, the starting point of our walk. We do this the next morning on a spotless local bus, chatting with passengers about the villages through which we'll be walking. Along the way, we get our first views of thatch-roofed cottages in storybook settings. How many times do I say the word "charming"?

In Chipping Campden, we take a photo of a stone that marks the start of the Cotswold Way. At the end of a leisurely afternoon exploring a seventeenth-century market square, renovated alms houses, and a crafts center, we begin our walk.

Two miles along the trail, we arrive at a lovely B & B, where two peacocks announce our arrival. Mindful of the two feathered alarm clocks that will be waking us at dawn, we make plans for an early dinner with friends, who will be walking with us for three days.

Beyond Base Camp
Principles for Planning an Itinerary

What follows is a checklist of organizing principles that we use to help us put together an itinerary.

PRINCIPLE ONE: RATE x TIME = DISTANCE

Remember yawning at this formula in algebra class? Well, it's time to wake up and dust it off. Because R x T = D is the immutable law of walking.

Tinker with one value and the other two change. And not always in your favor. Reduce your rate of speed, for example, while going the distance you've set for the day, and you could arrive at your B & B well past teatime—after the biscuits (cookies) have been consumed.

I'm thinking about this formula at mile thirteen on the last day of our walk along the South Downs Way with three miles still to trudge. My motivation to keep going is a long-anticipated victory march into Winchester, followed by a hot bath. But I'm not a happy walker. About a mile back, I lost interest in my surroundings. Pleasure morphed into determination, joy into intensity. What remained of my "ah ha" spirit of discovery and my "oh, look at that" tourist enthusiasm had disappeared.

Mike, too, is weary. Our rate is slowing, our time lengthening, as R x T = D takes on new meaning. With the sun setting, "D" now equals descending blood sugar, demanding appetite, and dwindling good sportsmanship.

What, then, constitutes sensible daily mileage? The answer varies because "it all depends." On hilly days about eight miles may feel right. Following a seven-mile day, a thirteen-mile day may be okay. The day after we walk thirteen, ten seems like a good number. On average, a comfortable "D" for us is about eleven miles.

Unfortunately, guidebooks frequently divide walks into fifteen-to seventeen-mile days. This distance works fine if the weather is clear, you know where you're going, and you're carrying a very light pack. It also helps if you ignore the sights and enjoy sipping water through a tube attached to a hydration pack while you march forward, rarely stopping, chewing up the miles, along with your water tube. Perhaps we're a little slow, but for us a fifteen-mile day seems a bit "over the top," although, sometimes, circumstances conspire to make such long distances necessary.

What about a sensible speed for walking? This also depends. At home, unencumbered, and only mildly interested in my everyday surroundings, I average about three miles per hour. But on vacation we travel about two miles, or a little less, per hour. We prefer slower rates and shorter distances because we like having the time to check our maps and observe our surroundings. We like pausing to restore body and "soles." We like snapping photos, nibbling al fresco, and talking with fellow walkers. In short, we like taking time to play.

We've never viewed walking as a contest, although many British walkers do. (See "Competitive Walking" in Step Nine.) We're not interested in how far we can walk in a day or how fast we can cover an arbitrary distance. For us a holiday ramble is an experience in "less is more": less distance per day, more time to enjoy every detail.

TIP : 4.3 SETTING THE PACE

- Select an average daily distance that suits you. When in doubt, be conservative. Mike and I prefer walking an eight to thirteen-mile day—sometimes a little more, sometimes a little less.
- Travel at a speed that's comfortable for you.
- Don't overdo. Rambling is supposed to be a pleasure—not a competitive sport.
- When selecting a guided tour, choose one with average daily mileage that appeals to you.
- When planning your own walk, set the mileage for your first few days a little lower than your average mileage.
- Factor in terrain. Less distance and a slower pace make for happy walking on hilly days.
- Vary your daily mileage. Give yourself some early afternoons to explore, rest, and do wash. (See Principle Three.)
- Be realistic. Let your pace reflect the athlete you are now, not the one you once were or the one you would like to be.
- R x T really does = D. Too few miles a day and the distance you need to cover may not fit the time available for your holiday.

- Too many miles a day can turn sore spots into blisters and transform the joy of *stepping out* into the chore of dragging on.
- Set your own pace, and go your own distance on all the paths you travel.

PRINCIPLE TWO: INFORMATION BEFORE RESERVATION

Before proceeding, you'll need to consider some basic questions. Your answers will help you select a trail and find accommodations that suit your interests and pace.

- How many days out of your total vacation are you planning to walk?
- How many miles would you like to average per day? Will this allow time for photo-ops, sightseeing, and visiting with other walkers?
- What time do you want to arrive at your destination each night?
- How do you feel about hills?
- Is there a special kind of scenery or historic period that beckons you?
- Can you schedule your travel off-season in cooler weather to avoid crowds?

TIP 4.4 LOCATING BASIC INFORMATION

(For more details, see Step Fourteen.)

- For general information and to get started, contact Visit Britain (previously, the British Tourist Authority). Call their office in New York City, or reach them on-line.
- An excellent source of information for the walker is the Ramblers' Association. Telephone them, or visit them on-line to request trail and accommodation guides, along with other items, facts, tips, and references that make planning a walk easier.
- Many trails, paths, and ways have their own websites.
- There are more than fifteen national trails in England and another fifteen in other parts of the British Isles. In general, more information is available on national trails than on trails maintained by local associations. A national trail is a good choice for a first walk.
- We like using national trail guides, accommodation guides, and trail strip maps to plan our walks. (Strip maps depict

a trail, roughly centered on a series of pages, and show features within a mile or so of a route.) These items can be ordered on-line or by phone and are excellent tools for planning a walk from overseas. (See Step Eleven, "Trail Guides.")

- Ordnance Survey, the national mapping agency of Great Britain, offers maps at various scales that are useful for planning and navigating, and can be ordered in advance. But you may need several of them, and they are not light.

When you've gathered your information, you're ready to get to work. Divide the trail you've selected into reasonable daily units, and begin making reservations. Use your handy accommodations guide, contact local tourist information centers, or locate your lodgings on-line.

TIP : 4.5 MAKING RESERVATIONS

- Decide how many miles you'd like to walk each day. Don't rush your journey. You're on vacation.

- Consider scheduling a day of rest or a few days of low mileage.

- Book your reservations from the States in advance, as we do, to prevent the hassles and frustrations of doing so en route.

- The spontaneous rambler may prefer to omit advanced reservations off-season on less popular paths. We are not spontaneous ramblers.

- Reservations are essential on all trails during summer months in a land where rambling is a passion.

- Some villages offer a tempting selection of accommodations. But in more remote locations, you'll have little or no choice. The one B & B that's there is the one you'll get—if you're lucky. Many remote accommodations will pleasantly surprise you. Some, of course, will disappoint. But you won't care, because your accommodations will be clean and dry and located where you want to rest.

TIP : 4.6 THE RIGHT ROOM FOR YOU

Overnight accommodations come in many shapes, sizes, and styles. And they all include breakfast! The most common selections—the ones you are likely to make—are listed below.

- Single: A room with one bed. Sometimes this is a double bed.

- Double: A room with a double bed. The rate for one guest in this room will be lower than for two because two guests use more towels and consume an extra breakfast.

- Twin: A room with two beds, usually two single beds, or one single and one double. The room rate is greater when two guests occupy a twin. Two beds make small rooms appear even smaller.

- Family room: A large room with beds that accommodate at least three people. Convenient for friends and families who enjoy each other's company and the luxury of a spacious room.

- Shared bath: The toilet and/or bath or shower will not be in your room. You will share these facilities with other guests. Usually not too many guests. This arrangement is not as inconvenient or as intrusive as it sounds.

- Private bath: The toilet and/or bath or shower is not in your room, but no other guests will share these facilities.

- Room with a basin: All of the above room configurations are greatly enhanced when they include a sink in your bedroom for your exclusive use.

- En suite: A room with all facilities in, or attached to, your room. Sometimes these will take the form of a lovely, modern bathroom. Other times, a shower stall, like a closet with running water, will be located inside your bedroom and will steam up your room when used. Your basin may be on a wall next to the telly (TV). And your toilet may be inside a separate tiny enclosure. But these facilities will be private and all yours. En suite arrangements are becoming more common and modern to suit today's tourists, who expect greater comfort and convenience than did the hearty travelers of the past.

One-of-a-Kind B & B—Dales Way

At 1,460 feet, where the Dales Way crosses the Pennines, we discover one of the highest farms in the Yorkshire Dales. A cluster of buildings located along a first century Roman road, Cam Houses marks the location of a settlement listed in the Domesday Book, England's first general census (1085–1086), conducted by order of William the Conquerer. When viewed from the outside, the sturdy stone dwellings do not promise much comfort, but Cam Houses divides what could have been a seventeen-mile slog over the spine of England into two days of more agreeable distance. We are relieved to have reservations here.

Our welcome, however, is not what we expect. On a small patio overlooking the distant hills, I remove my boots, setting them aside to air and dry, while our hostess bustles off to prepare tea. When I look up, eight sheep, driven by a young, overeager border collie, are racing in my direction. They stampede across the patio, over my boots, and through the front door, which, as is the custom in almost all weather, has been left open to invite in fresh air. The commotion rejuvenates Sue, a retired sheepdog resting inside. Rushing to assist our shouting hostess, and in obvious ecstasy, the old-timer turns around the bleating intruders in the hallway and chases the wooly mob back out the door before I have time to remove my boots from a second assault. Not the method I would have chosen for breaking them in.

In this remote setting, we spend a near-perfect evening. Our room is clean and comfortable. Mrs. S provides extra towels, a space heater, and a hair dryer. She even dresses for dinner (a three-course feast), as does her partner, a classic Yorkshire man, who raises sheep as generations before him have done. But not, he says, as generations after him are likely to do.

We think about the predicament walkers will encounter in this high, open country if these special people sell their farm and close their B & B. We know we've been fortunate to have stayed here. In the morning when we say good-bye, we sense that we are leaving a traditional way of life behind.

Note: I have since learned that Cam Houses continues to operate as a B & B under new ownership.

Principle Three: Rest Stops Matter

Even God rested. And so do we, although not necessarily on the seventh day.

We take our first day of rest before we begin a walk. We rest for another day at the end to celebrate. And we select at least one nice location for a pause along the way.

We pause by walking a half-day and checking into our B & B early, then hanging out for a long afternoon. We use our free time to rest and repair our body parts. We write postcards, apply waterproofing to our boots, and wash clothes. If we're in a village, we enjoy browsing, shopping, eating, and visiting tourist sites.

During our afternoon off, we might indulge in afternoon tea, as we did halfway along the Coast to Coast Walk in a tea shop on the town green in Reeth. With trays of pastries before us, we lingered more than an hour before venturing out in the rain to purchase a sand-casting of a border terrier, which we mailed home from the local post office. It greets us now each morning from a windowsill in our kitchen, a reminder to save some time each day to sit awhile and enjoy a nice cup of tea.

We also spent an afternoon in a quiet pub in Llanymynech on the Offa's Dyke path, slurping up pasta covered in thick homemade sauce while we watched a cricket match on TV and listened to our companion, Robin, laying bare the basics of a game as hard to crack as the Enigma Code. Cricket, like a foreign language, is best learned when one is young.

On a free afternoon in Grassington on the Dales Way, I dallied over a memorable warm goat cheese salad before visiting the local shops. In Kings Stanley on the Cotswold Way, I rested in the stillness of an English perennial garden, while Mike took a nap in our room and our laundry fluttered in the wind.

Now, on stressful days, my mind returns to these villages and gardens. Remembering them restores my resolve and recharges my energy. In their quiet places, I gather strength. And from them, I move forward again.

Full Day at Leisure—Coast to Coast Walk

On longer journeys, we schedule a full day of rest in addition to several early afternoons. We do this somewhere beyond the midpoint of the trail, on the psychological "downhill" portion of our journey. Stopping for an entire day, spending two nights in one place, is not as easy as it sounds. A day off alters routine and, at first, feels like a waste of time. Most walkers prefer to keep moving.

I am feeling this way when we arrive in Richmond, a charming Yorkshire town with shops, eateries, and cobbled streets. Located on the Coast to Coast Walk, it is a community with its very own castle, a restored Georgian theater, and a helpful tourist information office.

We've been walking for eleven, mostly dry, days. We've trudged over peaks in the Lake District and across hills and dales in Yorkshire. Easier walking in the fertile Vale of Mowbray lies ahead. Richmond seems like a perfect location for a day of repose.

But we are dubious. Last night we shared a farewell dinner with David and Sheila, whom we met on a mountain peak a week ago. After several days of walking together, including some time shared searching for the correct footpath, we've become friends. Now they are leaving us, moving on tomorrow. They wish they could indulge and take an extra day to rest, but they have a schedule to keep. We wish we could go forward with them, but feel we need a break. Finishing a day ahead of us, perhaps they'll walk in sunshine. Perhaps not. One day can make a difference in fickle weather.

We try to convince ourselves that a rest day is not a waste of time, that it is essential. My journal entry seems to confirm this.

== ❦ Journal ==

Losing It

Today it came to me, as we enjoyed thick soup in a cozy tea room, that this trip is too long, and that I want very much to have it done. It's become more chore than joy. Too much effort for too little pleasure. I'm getting tired of playing the role of "sweaty, good sport." ❧

The next morning our packs lean against the wall of our spacious bedroom, which overlooks a backyard garden. Our laundry is done, our mail ready for the post, and a full English breakfast awaits. The day is bright.

Trying not to dwell on the fine weather we're "wasting" while marking time in place, we set off to explore Richmond.

Light as crabs that have shed their shells, we fly pack-free down one Richmond hill and up another until we arrive at a narrow staircase that leads to the top of the castle wall and a glorious view of town and country. We descend to the great hall where we imagine knights gathered at a banquet, tossing table scraps to wolfhounds curled up on the stone floor.

We also visit the Georgian theater, picturing ourselves at a performance. We strain to hear the actors above the din of a rowdy audience in the days when English citizens in the American colonies were challenging the laws of King George III.

We visit Richmond's pharmacy where we each purchase the "just in case" knee and ankle supports we have carried ever since.

Our purchase is inspired by two youthful American ramblers. When we met them, they were hobbling on painful, unreliable knees, which they had wrapped inadequately in makeshift bandages. Of course, they'd been tramping fifteen to twenty miles a day, which may have had something to do with their knees rebelling and giving out.

A luxurious afternoon nap revives us, and we look forward to an early dinner at a small French restaurant. I'm considering the option of settling in Richmond permanently or, at least, of forsaking the next seven days of walking to Robin Hood's Bay. Time off is so civilized, so pleasant, so seductive!

Surprisingly, it is not difficult to get going the next morning, which turns out to be sunny after all. We have no regrets about "wasting" yesterday. With our knee and ankle braces safely stored in our packs and with our energy and spirits restored, we resume our march to the North Sea.

Full Day to Explore—Offa's Dyke Path

Relaxation is not an issue when, two years after our C-to-C walk, we stop in Trevor on the Welsh border. We know we need a day off. We've been walking for fourteen days and have four challenging ones ahead. We are ready for a change of pace. And we get a grand one.

David and Sheila have driven up from Nottingham to spend two days with us. We last saw them in Richmond on the Coast to Coast Walk when they "carried on" while we stopped for a day of rest. We've exchanged letters for two years and are looking forward to a reunion and to introducing them to Robin, our current walking companion. They will spend two nights at our B & B and have planned a day of sightseeing for us in the countryside of Wales.

Our day off dawns raw and rainy. No deluges, but a good day to be seeing sights from inside a car, with a driver who has cycled and walked on holidays in Wales. We visit Caernarfon Castle, the site of Prince Charles's investiture as Prince of Wales. We walk about its walled town, stopping for tea (of course) and driving on to a community with the distinction of having the longest name in Great Britain.

Three local women stop to help us pronounce its tongue-tying combination of letters: lanfairpwllgwyngyllgogerychwyrndrobwllllllantysiliogogogoch, which they tell us means, "The Church of Mary in the Hollow of the White Hazel near the Fierce Whirlpool and the Church of Tysilio by the Red Cave." Spitting and giggling, the five of us try to imitate the experts. We don't come close. Welsh is not for sissies.

After dinner I sit with Sheila, who has brought a photo album of their Coast to Coast Walk. She assures me I will complete this journey as well. Sitting quietly next to her, enjoying her support, I am aware that, although I have the world's two best travel mates, I miss having a girlfriend along. It isn't that I mind stopping with "the boys" to identify every airplane overhead. It's just that, for me, girl gossip is so much more engaging.

The next morning, our host snaps a group picture: five friends from different places who share a love of walking. David and Sheila drive off, vowing to return to walk the Offa's Dyke Path themselves. Mike, Robin, and I head off in our slickers. Up ahead the sky is clearing.

TIP : 4.7 IDEAS FOR A GETAWAY DAY

· Rent a car

· Borrow a bike

· Barge on a canal

· Hire a cab

· Take a bus

· Ride a horse

- Read a book
- Sit in a garden
- Take a walk
- Explore a museum
- See the sights
- Visit the shops

Principle Four: Overseas Connections

Listings in accommodation guides include complete addresses, details about available rooms and services, phone numbers, and grid references, which locate a listing with great precision on a map. A few will include a website. Many will have an e-mail address. We make our reservations by telephone. Here's how and why:

- We begin by signing up for our phone company's international plan. Spending fewer than ten cents a minute, we feel free to take the time we need to discuss our reservation with our future hosts.
- On the phone we get to hear about available rooms before selecting, sight unseen, the one—or the en suite combination—that most appeals.
- Making phone calls tells us our fate immediately. If no room is available, we ask the people rejecting us to recommend another B & B, which they almost always do. Perhaps a neighbor has a room. If she does, we call the neighbor and take our chances. This has worked well for us, and it is a good way to discover accommodations that are not listed in a guide.
- It is critically important to get explicit directions from the trail to your lodgings. This is best done by direct phone contact. To avoid confusion, have your trail map in hand when you call.

Tip : 4.8 Grandma Doesn't Have a Website
- The Web is not always the best resource for locating lodging and making reservations along a path.
- The Web is most useful for booking rooms in cities and towns because many communities list their accommodations on-line.

- The Web is also useful for locating fine lodging. The more upscale and pricey the accommodation, the more likely it is to have its own website.

- Traditional, small, and personal B & Bs, located in the countryside close to a path, are more difficult to uncover. They are mainly the private residences of individuals who have extra bedrooms because "the children have left home." These B & Bs are not likely to have their own websites, although many will have an e-mail address.

- Accommodation guides are available for national trails. (See Step Fourteen for more information.) These handy guides are better than "free range" Web searching for locating B & Bs. We use them as often as we can.

Principle Five: Confirming Reservations

Confirming a reservation is an art form. One of its major functions is to reassure a host who views you as a risk. You are, after all, an unknown from overseas. In most cases, you will not be sending a deposit, and your credit card will be useless. This is why you need to mail or, as is becoming more common, e-mail a confirmation.

Tip : 4.9 Confirmation Basics

Wait until you've made all your reservations before you send out confirmations. Be sure to confirm every reservation. The basic elements to include in a confirmation are:

- dates of arrival and departure

- the number of nights you will be staying

- the type of room you are reserving (twin, double, en suite)

- special requests for breakfast. We ask for porridge (oatmeal).

- lunch arrangements, if you'll be taking a box lunch with you in the morning. We rarely do. We prefer snacking. (See Step Eight.)

- dinner preferences if you're having an evening meal at your B & B. Whenever we can, we eat in. Home cooked meals en route are usually excellent. (See Step Eight.)

- a request that your host make a dinner reservation for you at a local pub or restaurant if she thinks you'll need one
- other special requests, such as for laundry and hair dryer use, driving you to and from dinner, picking you up from a point on the trail, or transferring your luggage
- the name of the B & B where you will be staying the night before your arrival. If your hosts start to worry (or are thinking about letting your room to someone who has just called), they can make a local phone call to the proprietor of your last B & B to check on your progress and receive assurance that you are very nice and on your way. In fact, we find it a common practice for hosts to check on guests in advance of their arrival.

Below is a confirmation letter we forwarded via e-mail to a B & B in Knighton. It is typical of those we send. I have also included the correspondence that followed. For convenience, and because it is more easily understood, when I write to confirm arrangements, I refer to Mike as "my husband," rather than "my companion."

Dear Mrs. S:

I am writing to confirm a reservation that my husband recently made by phone. It is for the night of Wednesday, 03 September, for an en suite family room for two adults.

We will leave the U.S. on 24 August. Until then, you can reach us by telephone at xxx or by e-mail at yyy.

We will be walking the Offa's Dyke Path. The night before our stay with you, we will be staying with Mrs. Helen V at xxx, Discoed, Presteigne, Powys LD8 2NW (Tel: yyy).

For your information, our favorite breakfast is juice and/or fruit with a variation of a full English breakfast: baked beans on toast with grilled tomatoes and mushrooms (when available). We prefer to omit eggs and sausages. Another breakfast we enjoy is hot oat porridge (made with water, rather than cream or milk).

And, especially, if the weather is cool or damp, we would love to have a warm bedroom for our arrival—or a space heater that we could turn on for a short time to warm the room. I get very chilly as I cool down after walking.

We look forward to spending the evening of 03 September with you and to getting back to Great Britain for our fifth walk!

Sincerely
Name and Full Home Address

———————————————

Dear Eleanor,

Thanks for your e-mail.

I confirm that I've reserved our en suite family room for you and your husband for 03 September as requested. I'll make sure the room is warm when you arrive. In addition to the central heating, there's also a room heater in the bedroom and one in the en suite shower room, so I'm sure you won't be cold.

No problem for breakfast—there are breakfast order forms in guests' rooms to complete, and all the items you mention are on the list. So you can choose exactly what you want when you're here.

We look forward to seeing you when you arrive on 3rd September.

Happy walking!

Regards,
Pat S

———————————————

Dear Pat,

Thank you for your reassurance about the heater. It's nice to know I will not be cold.

We look forward to seeing you on 03 September and hope you'll send along some good weather to greet us.

Best regards,
Eleanor Berger

Best Made Plans Go Awry

On a rest day at the end of a two-week ramble, after three hours of train travel, we arrive in Exeter in the early afternoon. With packs on our backs, we trudge uphill from the station, weary and looking forward to dropping our belongings at our B & B. We are planning to spend what's left of the sunny afternoon exploring the historic, university town.

The door of our B & B is opened by Nina, a twenty-something female who manages the establishment for an owner who is not at home. We have reserved a twin en suite, but Nina cannot find a record of our reservation. She apologizes profusely, explaining that her B & B is full, and it is likely that all other accommodations will be full as well. It is the Saturday night of student orientation weekend, and "no vacancy" signs are everywhere.

"Well," I say, "we have nowhere else to go. Please find us a room. Any type of room. We don't have a mobile phone and would not know whom to call if we did. We'll just rest here on your stairs while you search."

Fortunately, the eighth B & B Nina phones has had a cancellation for a double with a shared bath. And best of all, it's just a short walk from where we are. We take it with relief and gratitude and tell Nina that she is our hero.

How could this have happened? Nina says that owner Arlene forgot to write our names in the all-important "book." But we know better. We've heard about unscrupulous hosts, who, given an opportunity to rent a room for several nights, simply erase the reservations made for one-night stays. They never bother to tell their abandoned guests. Nor do they find another room for them. This is an especially onerous practice when its victims are tired walkers.

We have heard about this, but we do not believe it until now. After more than one hundred comfortable nights in British B & Bs, this is the first time we have encountered such mean-spiritedness. And, it appears, there was nothing we could have done to prevent this from happening.

Before leaving home we phoned Arlene twice, once to make our reservation and once to get specific walking directions to her B & B from the station. We reserved our room with a VISA card. We confirmed the room by e-mail, and Arlene sent a confirmation e-mail to us in return. She had five opportunities to remember to put us in the "book."

Could this happen again? Yes, but it's unlikely. Only one chance in a hundred. But the experience is a reminder that in spite of one's best efforts, best laid plans do go awry—and that good people like Nina are there to help when they do.

Principle Six: Managing Public Transportation

We depend on public transportation (trains and buses) to take us to our destinations. This is a treat for us, living as we do, in a nation that neglects its own public transportation options. Mike spends time visiting the National Rail Enquiry Service on-line and conversing with BritRail clerks on the phone. (See Step Fourteen for more information.) Still, we have made plans based on what we thought were the best available train times, only to discover that there were better choices. This is because the most reliable information about fares, routes, transfers, and times of departures and arrivals is available on location. We now finalize the details of our travel schedule after we arrive in country.

Tip : 4.10 Tickets and Schedules

· Don't get discouraged. Deciding when, where, and how to purchase train tickets is not for the faint-hearted. Only natives—and not all of them—are capable of sorting out the options offered by BritRail. Just "give it a go," and do the best you can.

· Arrange for your rail passes before you leave the States. Many discount passes, good for several days of travel, are only available when purchased from overseas.

- Check on coach (bus) and train schedules when you pass through a station on the way to your lodgings. Do this as soon as possible after you arrive, when you have the time and don't have a train or bus to catch.

- Ask a helpful window clerk for advice on the easiest and least expensive way to get to where you're going. If this requires queuing up, do it anyway. Reading or chatting while you wait in a queue helps time to pass quickly.

- Information obtained on-line is not entirely reliable. It often changes. We have saved time, money, and frustration by rechecking our information on location.

- Buy tickets and reserve seats (if advised) in person at a station a day ahead if you can. This helps to significantly reduce ticket cost and personal stress.

- Arrive at train and coach stations early.

- Buy your lunch before boarding. Selections at the station will be better than the offerings on the train.

- You'll have more fun when you take your time, make certain all is well, and get a good night's rest.

Whew! That's Done

With less than a month to go, it's time to gather our travel gear into a "staging area" and begin the process of shaking down and weighing in. For this we proceed to Step Five and some thoughts on final preparations.

Step 5

Getting Set
The Countdown

"Getting there is as important as being there."
LAO TZU (CIRCA 500 BCE)

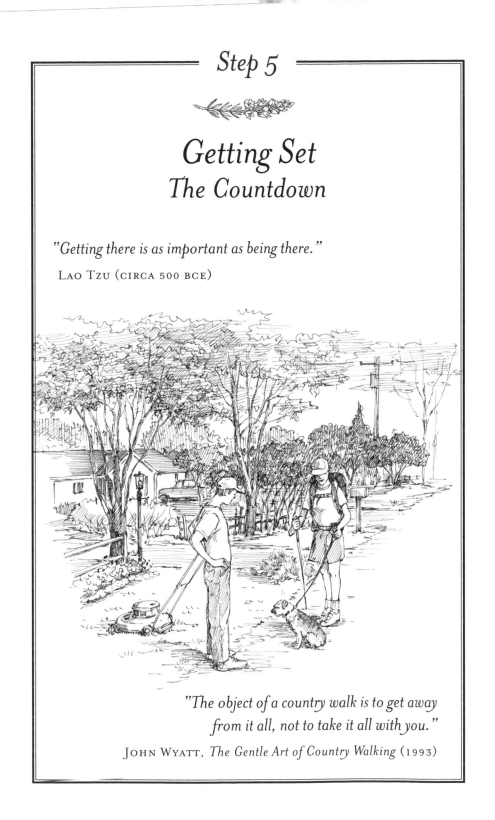

*"The object of a country walk is to get away
from it all, not to take it all with you."*
JOHN WYATT, *The Gentle Art of Country Walking* (1993)

Three Weeks to Go: Shakedown

Editing

Redundancy

Debate

Who Says?

Advice

Friendly Fire

Tip 5.1: Filtering Advice

Inquiring Minds

Tip 5.2: Folks Will Be Asking

Weighty Matters

Tip 5.3: Burdens Are Relative

Taking Care

Tip 5.4: Keeping Whole and Healthy

Two Weeks to Go

Journal: Second Thoughts

A Note from Mike's Mother, Louise

Dear Friends

Tip 5.5: Measures of Success

One Week to Go

Dress Rehearsal

Magic Moments

Come Along

Three Weeks to Go: Shakedown

EDITING

Our living room has been transformed into a staging area. Our sofas are covered with gear, clothing, and incidentals. I have claimed the three-cushion one as mine, leaving the smaller two-seater for Mike. And therein lies the problem. Whenever he walks by my collection of stuff, he begins his mantra: "Every ounce counts," adding, "Time to lighten up. Look how much less I have on my sofa."

Hearing this, I feel guilty—and a little panicky—about my pile. Will it fit into my pack (which seems to be shrinking the closer we get to launch day)? Will I be able to carry it for six hours a day? Why didn't we sign up for a tour or luggage service?

Gazing at my sofa and seized by Mike-induced anxiety, I retreat to a mantra of my own: "Edit, girl. Edit. Remove redundancies." But which of my treasures is redundant?

Yesterday, I removed three bandannas from my sofa. This morning, however, I replaced the one with an orange/blue/kelly green print because it goes nicely with the olive green nylon shirt I plan to wear every evening—and which will become very boring if I don't accessorize it once in awhile with a touch of color.

I also added a perky, pink, absorbent, jogger's headband to replace the second bandanna. So let's see: three items, minus three, plus two, equals minus one bandanna. Good for me. My pack feels lighter already.

REDUNDANCY

Today I'm stuck on socks. I circle my sofa, staring at three pairs for rambling and an extra one for evening use. Do I need all four, or do I only want them? Do I want them enough to carry them on my back for a hundred miles? Of course, I'll be wearing one pair. That leaves only three to carry. Not bad.

"Take the risk, and leave one of the extra pairs behind," urges a deep inner voice (probably Mike's). "You'll find places to wash your socks. You'll find ways to dry them. They're not going to wear out. Go ahead. Two extra pairs are enough. Ounces count."

I stop circling and remove one pair from my pile. I lay them on a nearby coffee table. Maybe I'll return them to the sofa later. But for now, they're out of bounds. I leave them there and walk away.

Debate

Mike and I seldom argue and never over small things—at least not without a reason. Today's reason is toothpaste.

Our antique butter bowl, which could serve salad to twelve hungry vegans, is filled with essential incidentals, which are spilling onto the dining room table: tissues, hand wipes, batteries, first-aid supplies, and film.

To eliminate "ounces that count," we have to sort through these. We decide to take all the film, but not the canisters. We agree to take more tissue packs and less lamb's wool, more upset stomach medicine, and less vitamin C.

When we get to toothpaste, civility deteriorates. Mike wants to know why I need two mini-tubes when he's taking only one. He suggests I remove half of my reduced supply. Eventually, and after several of his snide remarks, I acquiesce, aware that we share the same dentist, and that I'll be reporting this incident when we return, and Dr. N is drilling my new cavities.

I reach into the butter bowl and remove one of the tiny tubes. Another two ounces lifted from my pack. Unless I put them back tomorrow.

Who Says?

Motto of a what-if person: "Better to have it and not need it, than to need it and not have it."

Motto of a happy walker: "Better to have it. But only if you need it and can carry it."

Advice

The closer I get to tramping a footpath, the more advice I receive from well-intentioned friends, many of whom have never done any rambling.

Judy, for example, suggests that I carry a pocket poncho, a garment that serves her well on canoeing and kayaking excursions. In fact, she is so certain that a poncho is critical to the success of my walk and the buoyancy of my spirits that she makes a special trip to our house to hand me one from her own collection. Her poncho now rests atop my waterproof, Gor Tex® jacket. It reminds me of a generous friend and an act of kindness, but is not likely to accompany me across a windy moor.

Nancy swears by her leather and fabric boots that have a waterproof liner. "I wouldn't walk anywhere without them," she says. Susan is equally attached to her traditional leather ones. She coats them with waterproofing and says she trusts them to carry her anywhere. I listen to both friends, but stay with the boots I bought. (See "Selecting Boots" in Step Two.)

Marilyn is a golfer whose idea of adventure is walking the links. She is trying to understand why I plan to walk a longer distance. She wants to know if I'm doing this of my own free will. She worries out loud about all the things that could go wrong. I remind her that Mike and I are not climbing K-2 and that walking is considered "soft adventure."

Still, to ensure the success of our journey, she hands me a small, red ribbon. "Carry this, and don't you dare forget it. It's for warding off evil spirits." The instant I grasp it, I feel stronger, safer, braver. Trust me. You don't want to travel without one.

My friend, JoAnne, qualifies as a guru. When she talks, I listen. She has walked in England and knows which "stuff" to pack. She recommends that I take several "just in case" items: repair tape, panty liners for days between laundry days, and a large plastic bag for storing wet things and for sitting on when the ground is damp. In this case "just in case" makes sense. I add her suggestions to my pack.

I love my opinionated, uninhibited friends and welcome their clarity and honesty, their thoughts and concerns. Now, however, as I step out of the familiar to walk new trails, I sense it is time to follow my own heart.

Friendly Fire

Not all friends say the right things. And those who do, don't always say them at the right time. This reality calls for selective listening because how friends view themselves and feel about risk can color their advice and well-wishes.

Tina, for example, is calm and cool about my imminent adventure. She has no interest in doing a long walk herself, but understands my excitement. She should. We've been sharing each other's lives for five decades, and nothing one of us does or says surprises the other any more. I've learned to accept that when Tina is "hiking out" off a heeling sailboat, getting cold and wet, she thinks she's having fun. So, for her, the fact that I want to "hike out" in my own way—even in the rain—is no big deal.

Helen, however, worries—especially about my back. She can remember when we both had back problems. Her concern is making me nervous, eroding some of the tenuous confidence I've been gaining. I'm starting to wonder if the back I almost stopped worrying about will hold up under the challenge ahead. I guess there's only one way to find out.

Then there's Elaine, who talks a lot about injuries and tells me how difficult it will be to do what I am attempting. Elaine is not a confidence builder. I prefer JoAnne's advice. She walked most of the Coast to Coast path with a stress fracture and swears she would do it again.

As time grows short, the worries and concerns of friends can be contagious. So, sort out your friends' advice, screen your calls, and stay the course. You're almost there.

TIP : 5.1 FILTERING ADVICE

: · Listen to experts and to those who care about you.

: · Select advice that is helpful, and ignore the rest.

: · Follow your instincts.

: · Use your intuition.

: · Listen to your heart.

INQUIRING MINDS

I feel flutters of excitement as I move from planning to a recognition that I'm really going to be *stepping out*. I can imagine countryside trails, Yorkshire accents, pints of ale pumped from basement kegs. Just a few more weeks, and I'll have a footpath beneath my feet and a smile on my face.

With time compressing, I've been walking more miles, more often, with additional weight in my pack. Although somewhat inadequate, my training is as much activity as I can muster in the time I'm able to steal from other demands.

And, now, there's a new challenge. My outings require additional time because they've become more social. Before I started walking with a pack, neighbors I passed would simply wave, smile, and briefly comment on the weather, or on my wearing hiking boots instead of sneakers. A few might pause to greet my terrier, Gambit, who returns kindness with paws-up enthusiasm. Recently, however, almost everyone has been stopping me to ask questions.

It seems that inquiring minds want to know what I'm up to, while I want to know if I'll ever complete a daily walk on time again. And Gambit wants to know why he's become so popular.

I've never been inclined to broadcast our travel plans in advance because I'd rather people not know when our home will be unoccupied. When asked, I always try to be vague about these details. Now, I find myself talking about our intentions with relative strangers and curious neighbors. Wearing a pack, I've discovered, is like wearing a placard advertising one's impending departure.

So be warned. Pack practice elicits questions for which you'll need friendly answers.

TIP : 5.2 FOLKS WILL BE ASKING

: (Also see Steps One and Thirteen.)

: · Why are you walking with a pack?

: · Where are you going?

: · When are you leaving? (a question best left unanswered)

: · How long will you be away? (another question to avoid)

: · How much will your pack weigh?

: · How many miles will you be walking?

: · Why can't you take a long walk around here?

WEIGHTY MATTERS

I want to talk about weight. Not the chronic, stick-to-your-ribs kind most of us want to shed, but the kind we're about to place on our backs.

There's an old saying: "A pint's a pound the world around." This is more than information. It's a warning about just how heavy things really are. And it's a reminder that if a liter-size bottle of water weighs about two pounds, those gallon jugs of water, which we lift into our cars, weigh eight pounds each. So, if your pack weighs twenty-three pounds, your back will be bearing the weight of almost three gallons of water!

Mike assures me that three gallons of weight, well-distributed and secured in a properly fitted pack, will actually feel quite comfortable. But I'm skeptical. After years of lugging groceries and water from car to kitchen, his assurances sound too good to be true.

What does ring true, however, is his confidence in the power of distraction. "Once we're underway," he says, "you'll be so captivated by the countryside, you'll forget about your pack and the miles ahead. Under the spell of green vistas, country gardens, and tidy villages, you'll think of other things."

I'll be counting on this when I slip my pack onto my shoulders.

TIP : 5.3 BURDENS ARE RELATIVE

- They feel lighter as we grow stronger.
- They are easier to carry when we have support.
- They trouble us less when we're happy and distracted by sunshine and scenery on a journey we love.
- If we redistribute some of our burdens and eliminate others, we'll be able to carry what remains (or find a nice luggage service to help us).

TAKING CARE

The weeks before leaving are weeks to stay focused, as we scurry from one detail to another, feeling like we have "squirrels on the brain." Long lists of "have-to-do's" appear and shrink, only to regenerate. We find books we think we need to read. (We don't.) We discover things we still have to buy. (We might.) And we find ourselves walking less than we'd like. (We'll have to strengthen our muscles on the footpath.)

In busy times it's important to relax, to take care of our health, and to take the time we need for "making lists and checking them twice." Our goal is to reduce stress—the rush-around disease that compromises immune systems, increases carelessness, invites injury, and causes accidents, which are not always accidental.

Many accidents, in fact, are predictable events that occur because we're distracted, overwhelmed, or just too tired to think. They derail dreams and plans, striking when our bodies are in one place and our stressed minds in another.

In these final days, to avoid mishaps, we need to stay focused, alert, and on guard against the demons of pre-trip stress and hurry-up excitement.

TIP : 5.4 KEEPING WHOLE AND HEALTHY

- Look for loose carpets, unexpected steps up or down, potholes, and other hazards that turn ankles, stub toes, and twist knees.

- In summer, resist the temptation to go barefoot.

- In winter, unless you're a skater, stay off ice, or take your time—and bend your knees—when crossing it.

- Wear comfortable, low-heeled shoes to avoid blisters or injury. Every day. Everywhere.

- Watch where you're going. No tripping, stumbling, or falling allowed.

- Lift carefully, especially something hot from the oven.

- Drive mindfully. (This applies to your bicycle, too.) Try to anticipate the crazy things other drivers might do.

- Wash your hands well, often, and always before touching your face or your food—even if you don't think you've come into contact with contagious sniffles, sneezes, or coughs.

- Breathe deeply as often as you can.

- Move gracefully. Smooth is safer than tense. Fluid is safer than agitated.

- Do one thing at a time. You can multitask when you return.

- Focus on the present. Take care of tomorrow when it arrives.

Two Weeks to Go: Closing In

Second Thoughts

Can you become too aware of your own body? I think so. And I think I am. With only two weeks to go, I'm tuned into every ache and pain. Is today's muscle spasm a sign that, finally, I am shaping up? Or have I twisted or strained some vital ligament or tendon?

Maybe I shouldn't be doing a one-hundred-mile walk. Maybe I'm pushing myself beyond my limits. Maybe that's a good thing to do. Maybe I should stop worrying and start feeling excited. Maybe I should just relax. 🦋

A NOTE FROM MIKE'S MOTHER, LOUISE

"Hopefully, you're all packed, practiced, and in shape. Eleanor, dear, please relax. Whatever weather, whatever adventure occurs, you will face and fully enjoy or, if necessary, factor out.

"Enjoy. Enjoy. And play it safe." (Well, Louise is, after all, a mother.)

DEAR FRIENDS

My decision is behind me. I'm trying out adventure—something tempting, something wonderful, but something that's also a bit of a stretch, especially for the backs of my legs. Please, don't look dubious when you ask about our plans. It's too late for concern. Instead, cheer me, encourage me, and, whatever you do, don't bring up the subject of stress fractures.

I'm not, after all, off to summit Denali. I'm simply taking a walk over scenic hills, across lovely countryside, and through picturesque villages. Be assured that our journey will be a success however far we travel because the ways in which we measure success have changed. Our new definition is more about delightful moments than about goals and destinations, more about satisfaction than about achievement, more about a what-if worrier becoming a free spirit than about walking an entire footpath.

TIP : 5.5 MEASURES OF SUCCESS
- If we stay healthy
- If we forget about our blisters—or don't get any
- If we manage to arrive at our B & B each night without going astray too often
- If it doesn't rain every day
- If we make new friends
- If we go as far as we comfortably can
- If, at the end of our journey, we wish we could keep on going
- If, when we finish, we are looking forward to another walk

One Week to Go: Ready or Not

I don't think I'll ever be ready. Even if I cull my clothes and get my incidentals sorted, even if I compress them all into the confines of my pack, even if my "have-to-do" list shrivels down to zero things-to-do, I'm sure there will be something I've forgotten.

Lately, I've been wishing I could invent a walking simulator—one that can reproduce the experience of walking all day, day after day, with a full (but relatively light) pack. As it is, I won't know if I can go the distance until I try, since rambling is a learn-by-doing experience.

Today, I got as close to a reality check as I'm likely to get. With my friend Carole Anne along to encourage me, I walked seven miles carrying a fifteen-pound pack. In spite of concern about some mysterious aches and pains that could be—who knows?—fractures and sprains, I now know I can go this distance. I know my ankles can do it. My knees and hips can do it. And my shoulders and back can do it. I am a team of working parts.

What I don't know is how well my team will do carrying twenty or more pounds for ten or more miles every day for two weeks. We think we can do it in spite of less-than-perfect preparation. But we'll have to wait and see. We'll have to be cheerful and brave in confronting our unknown. And we can't remember ever having done that before.

Dress Rehearsal

Sporting a new quick-dry haircut, I'm dressed head to toe in my new lightweight performance duds. I'm walking; they're wicking; we're all breathing. For weeks I've been testing my foot gear. It seems solid and should serve me well.

Ditto for my hiking pants. We've walked many miles together, and I can vouch for them. No chafing, no binding—even after hours of road testing.

During last week's storm, I donned my rain gear for its final test. Gaiters, pack cover, and waterproof jacket all passed. I came home dry. My jacket, though, was a little scratchy on my bare neck. I'll have to wear it over a bandanna or a shirt with a collar.

Today I put on my long sleeve blouse and my long sleeve zip-up undershirt. I have never tested them in combination and I'm relieved to report that they fit nicely, breathe well together, and are loose enough on my wrists to accommodate my watch.

My pack straps are adjusted. Under each, I wear a folded fleece sock to protect my bony clavicles. Somehow the socks stay in place and prevent soreness. I can even use them in the rain because they dry quickly. And they will double as booties at B & Bs with cold floors. Very useful. Very cozy.

Testing different clothing combinations, however, turns up an unanticipated problem. Uncomfortable underpants. The culprit is a label on the inside of a waistband. When my pack rests on it, the label presses against, and scratches, my skin, which is quite raw. Not good.

Back home I remove the label, but its remnant still irritates my back. I don't have time to buy new "wickie" underpants. So I try tucking my undershirt between my red skin and the offending garment. Relief. Who would have guessed that testing one's underwear could save a walk?

A dress rehearsal? I wouldn't go on stage without one.

Magic Moments

There are moments on my daily walk when I'm entirely comfortable and confident, when I feel as strong as an athlete and as happy as a child. In these moments, I'm unaware of effort. I forget about deadlines. I block out traffic noise, muddy roadside shoulders, unsightly telephone wires, and the ugly, thoughtless structures that blight local landscapes. Seduced by motion and propelled by the spirit of walking, I'm unaware of discomfort, except for an occasional need to piddle—a hip belt's way of letting a mature walker know that it's got a tight hold on her.

As I tramp along, trying to ignore this mild urgency, butterflies of excitement fill me with anticipation. Practice time is almost over. The curtain is rising.

For us, opening night will be an overseas flight. And now, I can't wait to be on it.

COME ALONG

Okay, that's it. We're ready. We're set (I think). Let's take off for a nice, long walk.

Step 6

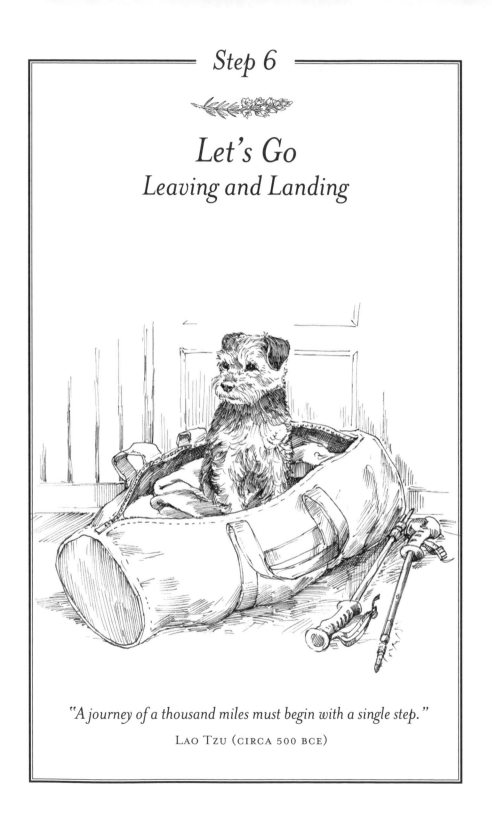

Let's Go
Leaving and Landing

"A journey of a thousand miles must begin with a single step."

LAO TZU (CIRCA 500 BCE)

Who Would Have Ever Dreamed?

With the Best of Intentions

Separation

Is This the Fun Part?

After a Night in Transit

Who Would Have Ever Dreamed?

Months of planning are laid out before me. Our living room is strewn with objects I never thought I'd be wearing or carrying in public. With less than a week to go before liftoff, I'm appalled that my list of "things-to-do" is still expanding. At this rate, I'll never reach its elusive bottom. Just this morning I added:

• run and unload dishwasher
• cancel newspaper
• give boots another layer of waterproofing
• distribute itineraries
• buy dog food to take to kennel

Travel, I'm learning, is a porthole through which we glimpse the experience of putting a life on hold. Its tasks and deadlines, plans and lists make me wonder how "Snowbirds" manage to shut down their northern lives and move their chilled bodies to Florida's warmer climes each winter. I marvel at how servicemen and servicewomen get up and go when duty calls, and how a woman like Sharon Lucid, at the age of fifty-three, was able to leave hearth, home, husband, and three children to live aboard Mir, the Soviet space station, for six months. She said of her adventure, "Who would have ever dreamed two years ago that I would be here?"

Indeed. And who would have ever dreamed two years ago that this "nervous Nellie" would be reviewing her own checklist, preparing to cut her ties with the familiar, readying herself to leave a warm house, easy-to-operate shower, and the comfort of sweatpants, mouthwash, and shaving cream for a three-week ramble across the British countryside? Who would have ever dreamed?

Certainly not my long-suffering father, who, some fifty years ago, was sharing an afternoon outing with his incorrigible ten-year-old daughter. The movie, *Singing in the Rain*, had just let out, and we were seated in a fancy little eatery.

Dad is suggesting I try something different from my usual fare. "The poached salmon looks good," he advises.

"Not to me," I assert. I'm holding out for my usual, a tuna salad sandwich.

"Look. The salmon won't hurt you. Try something new. Come on. Be adventurous."

"No, thanks. Not today."

New things and adventure hold no appeal. I order the tuna sandwich. My dad, who could persuade almost any jury to acquit almost any unsavory client, retreats in defeat.

Now, in my living room, surrounded by items selected for our walk, I hear my dad's voice again, urging me forward. "Come on," it is saying. "Be adventurous."

This time my reply is different. "Okay," I whisper. "I will."

It is five decades later, and I'm finally ready to "try the salmon." In fact, I'm looking forward to it.

Who would have ever dreamed?

With the Best of Intentions

Leaving for parts unknown and paths unexplored isn't easy. Confronting the unpredictable never is. I don't know—and don't think I really want to know if the health gods will watch over us, the map gods will guide us, or the weather gods will favor us. What I do know is that the days ahead will be different from any in my past. Perhaps enchanting, perhaps uncomfortable, probably both.

So, to my pile of new clothing and gear I'm adding a few rules, guaranteed to adjust attitude faster than a half-pint of ale at a local pub.

TIP : 6.1 RULES FOR ATTITUDE ADJUSTMENT

- When in Rome, I will do as the Romans do, even if I'm sure I know how to do it better.

- When I see a hill ahead, I will tell myself to "just get over it."

- I will express only half of my complaints and all of my delights.

- I will not share all of my suggestions.

- I will be a good sport most of the time and remain silent when I'd rather whine—if I can.

- I will expect to get wet.

- I will not worry about minor aches and pains.
- I will not overreact to "cold" and "thirsty." They are seldom fatal conditions on a countryside walk.
- I will not take detours and other inconveniences too personally.
- I will not worry. I'll try to remember that I'm walking for fun.
- I will view the experience as an opportunity to practice grace under pressure, even if I am tired, concerned, uncomfortable, and unable to control the variables of weather and terrain.
- I will not berate myself if I can't follow all of these rules.

Separation

Whether I'm strolling for pleasure or preparing for a holiday-on-foot, walking for me is a two-being exercise. I never walk alone. Sometimes Mike is with me. Sometimes Sara, Carole Anne, or Megan comes along. But, always, there is Gambit. In all seasons and in all weather, except the most extreme, he is by my side. Or, more likely, out in front challenging every cat or squirrel that dares to cross his path. He is all terrier, all the time: very game, very alpha, ever ready to get up and go.

Of all the things I yearn to take with me, but cannot, Gambit is the hardest to leave at home. I'm not sure I'll be able to walk without him. Sadness over our separation is deflating my happy anticipation.

Of course, Gambit is not making my imminent departure any easier. He's abandoned his daytime sleeping quarters (a soft woolen blanket draped across a king-size human bed) for my pile of hiking pants, T-shirts, and long johns, which he has formed into a carefully layered nest, guaranteed to wick away any trace of canine moisture. Occasionally, he raises his otter-like head to stare at me as if to ask, "Aren't you forgetting something?" Gambit is very good at guilt.

To avoid his gloomy gaze, I considered gathering and packing my gear just before departure. But a countryside walker needs to select and lay out possessions ahead of time to determine which favorite things to leave behind. Unfortunately, the dog nesting in my clothing happens to be one of them.

Pressured by his pathetic stares, I reassure both Gambit and myself that I am not abandoning him. On the contrary, he'll be a guest at Joan's exceptional kennel, staying with someone who treats her canine visitors like royalty. I remind him that he has vacationed there in the past and returns home as happy as a kid after a stay at Grandma's.

Gambit has removed himself now from my pile of clothing and is rubbing his oily flanks on my hiking boots and backpack, ensuring that a bit of him will travel with me. He stops to eye me suspiciously, puzzled by all my hugging and petting. I can't help myself. I miss him already.

As I gather my gear and prepare to separate from Gambit, I think about the little guy I'd like to take with me, the one eager to share my adventures. My walking buddy and plucky protector. My all-weather companion. The only "object" I already regret leaving behind.

Is This the Fun Part?

You've packed your gear. The living room is clear for the first time in a month. Your list of things-to-do is done. It's liftoff time at last.

Your trip to the airport is uneventful. You arrive on time, check in, and subject yourself to a security inspection that compromises personal space and privacy. Hours later, you board your flight and begin to relax. Your stress level drops from red to orange.

Trying to settle into your cramped seat, you ask yourself, "Is this the fun part?" For me, it isn't—at least not yet. An overnight flight in a sardine can is not my idea of fun. At night I prefer to sleep, which is why I carry an inflatable travel pillow. But on planes today I rarely doze, even with my pillow. Sleeping requires a modicum of leg and fanny room, and that doesn't exist in coach.

So I sit up thinking. First, about the disgruntled employees who did ground maintenance on a plane I'm trusting with my life, then about the luggage mafia, who, in theory, stowed aboard our precious duffel bag, but probably didn't. I'm not happy about the man crunched in next to me, who has a cold—or worse—that appears to be contagious. Nor do I feel nourished by microwaved meals served by overworked flight attendants, who resemble zookeepers tossing fish to sea lions. Flight-induced fatigue doesn't do much for my attitude.

Relief arrives at last. We land safely, pass through immigration, and proceed to baggage claim. And there it is waiting for us—our very own duffel. I silently thank the luggage mafia and apologize to the ground crew that serviced our plane. I am groggy, but excited. The fun part has begun!

TIP : 6.2 SURVIVING A FLIGHT IN STEERAGE

· To reduce jet lag, avoid dehydration. Drink plenty of non-alcoholic, decaffeinated beverages on board. Plane cabins are very dry.

· Walk about the cabin when you can. Climb over carts if you must.

· Get up and stretch every few hours. You'll find some space near the restrooms and emergency exits. If other passengers stare, ignore them. After you collect your luggage, you'll never see them again.

· Place the pillow provided by the airplane in the small of your back for support.

· Use a travel (neck) pillow for sleeping. (Inflatable ones are easy to pack.)

· Wear eye shades and earplugs to help you sleep.

· Drink coffee or tea with the meal/snack served before landing. It will perk you up for the day ahead and help reset your biological clock.

· Lower your travel expectations. Comfort in coach class is a thing of the past. Tell yourself that claustrophobic misery is a temporary condition you can endure and that it builds character.

· Focus your thoughts on the future and on the glorious days of walking ahead. The philosophy of "be here now, stay in the present" has its limits. Economy class is one of them.

After a Night in Transit

If you've flown overnight and slept poorly, the haze in which you arrive is not jet lag. It is sleep deprivation, and only sleep will cure it.

Our approach is to stay awake and to keep busy until dark, ignoring the fuzziness as best we can. We drink healthful fluids, eat light meals, and, after checking into our hotel, do some sightseeing, rain or shine. We avoid making important decisions and watch where we place our tired feet, especially when crossing streets.

After a full day of exploration, we have an early dinner and return to the hotel to sort out our belongings and prepare our backpacks for the day ahead. (See "Base Camp Alternatives" in Step Four.)

Usually, the long hours since we were last in bed, a busy day of sightseeing, and our relief that we are safe and sound are enough to reset our travel-weary bodies to local time. We feel grateful, relaxed, and almost always very tired. It may be late afternoon on the East Coast, but in our new home it is time to sleep, so that tomorrow we can go out and play.

A Soft Berth

On the day we arrive, I attempt to stay awake. (See Step Six.) No matter how jet lagged I feel, I try to wait until nightfall before I give in to sleep, confident that when I do, the bedroom in which I collapse will be like many others we'll inhabit in the weeks ahead. It will be clean. It will have challenging plumbing, sporadic heat, and fabulous comforters. It will be decorated in tasteful, coordinated fabrics. But it will not have flannels (washcloths), which is why we usually carry our own.

Whether we are staying at a hotel or inn, a pub or guest house, a youth hostel or farm house, the price for a night will include a "full English breakfast." This feature makes every accommodation a "bed and breakfast" and every B & B—whatever its shape, size, or condition—a British institution.

Like a spell of fine weather, the right B & B can transform an average day of walking into a day to savor and remember.

BEST BED AND BREAKFASTS

As I see it, the best B & Bs are not the most luxurious. Rather, they're the ones with the nicest, most nurturing, most approachable hosts.

We can manage for one night to live in a small room with knick-knacks on every surface and no space to set out our toiletries—as long as our host offers us a dryer or a warm space for hanging our laundry and wet clothes. It doesn't matter if we sleep in a bedroom with closets and dresser drawers so crammed with clothing that our belongings have to be piled on the floor—as long as our host asks if there is anything she can get for us.

It is fine with me if I have to share a bathroom and wear my eye glasses in the shower, because without them I can't read the complicated instructions for operating the hot water—as long as the facilities are clean and functional, and a thoughtful host has provided some of the little things that make showering pleasant: shampoo and soap, for starters.

It doesn't matter that hot and cold sink taps—even newly installed ones—are separate and extend only an inch or two over the basin, so that a contortionist would have a hard time washing up without scalding her hands or bruising her knuckles. One learns to wash carefully and carry one's own sink stopper for such contingencies.

What does matter is how welcome we feel and whether our comfort is important to our hosts—in short, whether we are treated like guests. When we are, we enjoy reciprocating by being especially good ones.

We take off our boots before entering, hang our wet things where we are instructed, leave our room in good order when we depart (even if only for dinner), and treat our temporary lodgings as if they belonged to us.

TIP : 7.1 GOOD B & B GUESTS

- Remember that they are staying in a private home
- Leave their boots and muddy gaiters at the front door
- Take care not to break the knickknacks in their room
- Ask if they can safely leave clothing on the radiator when they leave for dinner (on the unlikely chance that the heat will come on while they're out)
- Wash out the bathtub for the next guest
- Appear promptly for meals, especially for dinner if they're having an evening meal at their B & B
- Tell the host how much they enjoy and appreciate the food and service
- Ask for what they want, instead of whining about what's not offered
- Understand that things will not be the same as they are at home, or as pleasing as they might have been the previous night at "that lovely guest house"
- Are prepared to pay for their room in cash or traveler's checks in local currency
- Notify a proprietor as soon as possible if they need to cancel or change a reservation
- Enthusiastically praise and fuss over the family dog—and the children and garden, too—but especially the dog

Thanks for the Memories: B & Bs at Their Best

Mrs. S, Washington—South Downs Way

You offered us the use of your telephone, living room television, and your personal hair dryer. We stayed in your son's room, and from you we learned all about him. We felt like family.

Alan and Brenda L, Bampton—Coast to Coast Walk

You found us waiting on your doorstep when you returned from a family gathering. We had requested an evening meal, and you surprised us when you asked us to join you and your visiting relatives from Dorchester for dinner. We enjoyed veggies galore, homemade meat pie, and trifle before retiring to our spacious, comfortable room. We were fascinated to learn that we were staying in an outlying grange, built in 1480, which was associated with nearby Shap Abbey, and that our bedroom had been the base of the original bell tower. After an excellent breakfast, we left reluctantly, crossing an ancient packhorse bridge to rejoin our trail.

Mrs. Julie C, Cringle Moor, North York Moors—Coast to Coast Walk

As we approached your farmstead, I thought we might have made a mistake in selecting such a remote dwelling for our overnight. Its utilitarian features gave new meaning to the term "working farm," but, as we passed through your kitchen, spied freshly baked scones, and received a warm welcome, we knew we were in for a treat. Our room was as clean and comfy as any we have occupied. And the bathroom we shared with two other guests had a heater!

We enjoyed getting to know your young family and your Yorkshire neighbor, although we had to struggle to decode his accent. One suggestion, though: In the morning, when temperatures are in the fifties, you might want to keep your front door closed until after your guests have layered on their fleece.

Chris and Pam K-F, Appletreewick—Dales Way

At the end of our first day on the footpath, we relaxed on your patio in the setting sun, enjoying homemade biscuits with our tea. We met Jean, your neighbor, whose fortieth anniversary party you had attended at the town hall the day before. She carried with her a large piece of her anniversary cake, which she shared, along with delicious gossip about the event. We send you a special "thank you" for drying our clothing and for giving us a lift to and from the local pub. We feel lucky to have started our Dales Way walk with you.

Brian and Louise W, Kings Stanley—Cotswold Way

We remember your doting on us, asking more than once if we needed anything—a question seldom asked in other homes in which we have stayed. And we were pleased to tell you that, in truth, you had taken care of everything, including us.

Mike and Helen V, Discoed—Offa's Dyke Path

Our room was small, but you thought of everything a guest could wish for. You tried hard to please, and certainly did. Our lamb dinner was perfect, as was the haddock you prepared for breakfast. But what we remember most is our long afternoon visit with your family over tea in your living room.

Discoed's special feature is said to be St. Michael's Church, located on a sacred Celtic site, and the 5000-year-old yew tree that marks the church's entrance. But for us, your B & B will always be Discoed's most memorable attraction.

Alison and Paul M, Gladestry—Offa's Dyke Path

When we think of pure elegance and pampering, we think of Dyke House. In your beautiful home, we found washcloths, soft terry robes, heat when needed, and a room so lovely and comfortable we hated to leave, which is why we stayed so late chatting with you the morning of our departure. Because the pub was closed, you provided an evening meal, which was served in an elegant and serene setting. It was the best dinner of our entire journey. We thank you for your warmth and impeccable hospitality.

Mrs. Sue S, Sigwells—Uphill to Old Harry

You met us with a smile when we arrived at your farm, and your warmth continued throughout our entire stay. We hope we adequately thanked you for hanging our damp clothing over your kitchen stove, washing out our water bottles, making our dinner reservations, and then driving us to and from a pub some distance away. We enjoyed visiting with you in your kitchen after dinner where we learned about badgers, raising cattle, and the trials of being a racing jockey. Our wish as we departed was that we might have remained at Beech Farm for a few more nights.

THE BED AND BREAKFAST CHALLENGE

It's not easy to sleep in a different bedroom every night. Every pillow is a stranger. Every bed feels unfamiliar. The plumbing is peculiar. Light switches and bathrooms are never where you expect them to be. Hosts keep changing, along with their rules, customs, and expectations, making every night a new adventure.

After a dreary, raw day of walking, I collapse my hiking pole as we approach our B & B. Another test of adaptability awaits. I'm hoping for the best. Only six days of walking, and I'm growing weary of playing "sweaty, good sport."

Our host answers our knock. Unwilling to put my pack down in a puddle, I'm bearing its weight as I remove my boots and balance against her door frame, while she watches my antics, like a cat eyeing a bird. In sock-covered feet, I pad along behind her to our room. "Lovely," I say when we enter, before I march off to shut two open windows.

She tells us there is a kettle in our room (but no snacks that I can see) and prepares to abandon us to our cold cell. I want to be a good guest. I do not wish to appear spoiled or demanding. I wait for her to inquire if there is anything else we need that she can get for us. She does not inquire. So, in my friendliest voice, I ask, "Do you have a hair dryer I might borrow, and perhaps two old towels we could use for wringing laundry? I'd also appreciate an extra blanket."

Silence. Then, frigidity. And, finally, but without enthusiasm, "I'll see what I can do. Is that all?"

I decide not to push my luck by asking for biscuits or a snack. Instead, I muster my courage and reach for the B & B gold ring. As impudent as Oliver Twist asking for more porridge, I take a deep breath and request...a space heater!

I give her my word that I won't abuse it. I promise I'll use it less than an hour. I swear that I'll plug it in only to remove the considerable chill from our room now and, perhaps again, in the morning if we wake before she turns on the heat. I also offer to pay for the extra electricity.

Yes. She has a space heater. "But," she says, "you won't need it. I'll turn on the heat at five tonight, and it will stay on until eleven."

Unfortunately, this will be when we're at dinner, after I'm already chilled down to my wet underwear and have taken my shower. Our host, of course, doesn't need a heater because she and her family will be gathering for tea and dinner in a toasty kitchen, warmed by a large stove.

Twisting her cold knife, she adds, "I turn the heat on again at eight in the morning,"

"How thoughtful," I want to say. "By eight, I'll be up and dressed in layers, and the heat won't matter." I also know from experience that by then her front door will be wide open to invite in fresh, fifty degree air and to let out all that pesky heat she turned on.

The implication here is that something is wrong with me, that it's all in my head, that this soft American needs toughening up. "You know," says the wicked witch of the South Downs Way, "you catch colds when it's too warm indoors."

Discussing this with my jailer in a damp, unheated room, after a damp day of walking, with sweat condensing into icicles under my bra, I cannot abide her drivel. I've had enough. "No," I reply. "Heat does not cause colds. Viruses cause colds. You get colds from not washing your hands. You get colds when infected people sneeze on you. I haven't had a cold in two years. And I would be very grateful if I could have a space heater for our room. Do you think we might use yours for one night?"

Yes, she will get it for us. Mike offers to help. I've embarrassed him again, and he's looking for something placating to do. I, in contrast, feel relieved and reassured. Until I remember that tomorrow I may have to go through this routine all over again.

Comfy Cozy
An Open Letter to Bed and Breakfast Hosts from a Five Star Guest

It's three o'clock in the afternoon. My partner Mike and I are on the last mile of a long day of walking. We are wet, tired, and muddy. Through hazy drizzle, we can see the village where our B & B and a hot cup of tea await. We press our tired legs and mud-caked boots forward.

We are within two days of completing the two-hundred-mile Coast to Coast Walk, our third trek in England. On this journey, as on our other walks, we have stayed at youth hostels, guest houses, hotels, inns, pubs, and in the homes of friends. Most of our evenings in England, however—more than a hundred so far—have been at an institution that raises hospitality to an art form: the family-run British B & B. We believe our personal experience "sleeping around" qualifies us to comment on this unique form of accommodation, which has become our home on countryside walks.

B & Bs, of course, vary mightily. This fact makes each of them special. But it also makes us wonder as we approach a new door at the end of every day whether the B & B before us will provide the amenities that say "welcome" to a weary walker.

What follows is one walker's list of essential amenities that every bed and breakfast, seeking to provide a comfy, cozy home for a night, should offer.

The list, however, comes with a request for B & B proprietors. Before dismissing its suggestions as those of a comfort-loving American, please take some time to complete the following exercise. It will help place the ideas that follow in perspective.

On the next cold, rainy day, put on a twenty to twenty-five pound pack, and go out for a long walk. When you are sufficiently wet and tired, return to your own B & B. Take off your boots, and carry your pack to one of your guest bedrooms. Unpack it. Place your toiletries on the dresser or table there. Hang up, or stack, your dry clothes in the space provided. Hang up your wet clothes in the proper place. Remain in your bedroom to have your tea. Or enjoy a warm sitting room if one is provided. Take a bath or shower, and hang up your wet towel. Later, when you return from the pub, snuggle under the covers and read a book or write your journal. The next morning put on the clothes that were supposed to dry overnight.

Okay. Now here's that list of essentials:

· **A chair or bench near the front door, preferably in a sheltered area**

With a chair to sit on, visitors won't have to struggle to remove their hiking boots while leaning against a wall in their slickers, balancing on one leg. Nor will they form a wet heap on your hallway carpet, as they tug at their boots and try to maintain some dignity.

· **An outdoor clothesline with room for guest laundry in sunny weather**

By three PM in the spring and fall, only a few hours of sunlight remain for guests to wash and dry clothing they will have to wear or pack the next day. This gives a walker's wet clothing a greater claim to the outdoor wash line than your own sheets, towels, and family unmentionables. Without sufficient space to hang wet personal clothing, a walker is going to feel mighty guilty when she removes the family's not-quite-dry laundry from the line and replaces it with her own.

· **Space indoors for drying wet clothes after a rainy-day walk**

The best place for wet clothing that is peeled off a walker who arrives soaked through is either on an indoor line (preferably near a warm stove) or inside a clothes dryer. A walker without these choices cannot be held responsible if she resorts to draping wet things over the only drying spaces available—a curtain rod or antique wooden dresser, for example.

· **A place for unpacking dry things**

An empty wardrobe with clothes hangers is good. Wall hooks and pegs, where clothing can air out, are better. Empty shelves work well. Even a chair or two will do. Floors are not good. So, if that's the only place provided for a walker to empty her pack, she may decide to spread her things across your clean bedcover—at least until she gets under the cover herself. And you may not think a pretty counterpane is the best surface for ripe walking gear.

· A flat, uncluttered surface for setting out toiletries

A walker's pack doesn't have much in it, so she doesn't need a lot of space for little bottles and tubes. But she does need some. If none is available, she may have to move aside family heirlooms. When she does, she will try very hard not to break them. She will also try to return them to their proper places before she leaves. If she succeeds, you won't have to search for them.

· A hair dryer

This is a lovely extra for any walker who has lightened her pack by leaving her hair dryer and its bulky overseas adapter at home. After a six-hour walk, dry hair is as comforting as a fluffy duvet, especially when a walker has to venture outdoors again to the local pub for an evening meal. Be assured. Guests with warm, dry hair are nicer to have around than ones with cold, wet heads.

· A warm place to gather

At the end of a day, relaxing with a cup of tea or coffee and some biscuits is more agreeable in a warm bedroom or common room. As a walker dries off, she cools off, which is why a cozy room is so important. A comfortable living room, where guests can meet to exchange stories and share advice, is an especially welcoming feature.

· Some extras that walkers will appreciate:
- bedside reading lamps
- books or magazines
- biscuits or a sweet with afternoon tea
- packed lunches available
- laundry service
- a bar of soap (or washing gel and a flannel for applying it)
- shampoo
- extra towels and blankets left where guests can help themselves
- a heated towel rack for drying wet bath towels
- an enthusiastic, nurturing host with time to chat and information and encouragement to offer

There is one "problem," however, for walkers who do manage to find a B & B with these amenities. When they enjoy such comforts in the evening, it may be difficult for them to depart in the morning.

And word gets around. Satisfied guests are certain to talk about their experience with other walkers seeking a "comfy cozy" B & B. Perhaps one just like yours.

The Youth Hostel Alternative

THINGS I'VE LEARNED ABOUT YOUTH HOSTELS

Eventually, almost every walker spends a night in a youth hostel (YH)—either because the distance between available B & Bs is too great, and a YH is the only option, or because a walker *prefers* to stay in one.

YHs are relatively inexpensive and clean. They offer an evening meal on location. The camaraderie is pleasant. And you get to stay with other girls or guys in a room that will bring back memories of nights spent at summer camp.

If you've seen one YH, you have not seen them all. They vary dramatically. At St. Briavels, for example, on the Offa's Dyke Path, we stayed in a small castle that some eight hundred years earlier had been one of King John's hunting lodges. Our dinner was a rollicking medieval banquet. Guests dressed in period costumes, which they borrowed from two sturdy, wooden trunks that looked ancient enough to have once contained King John's tunics.

On the South Downs Way we stayed at Tottington Barn Youth Hostel, a rambling, converted 1930s summer house. It was clean and run according to the rule book. Men slept in a dorm room separate from women. Never mind that there was only one other gentleman guest and several rooms that Mike and I might have shared. Those rooms were designated "women only" and not available for couples. Dinner was somewhat edible. We washed the dishes, hoping that the guests before us had washed ours with as much soap and care. We slept well on our bunk beds tucked inside lovely comforter-like sleeping bags that had fresh liners, which we returned the next morning for laundering.

- You will meet guests of all ages, especially active seniors off-season.

- Guests sleep on bunk beds in family rooms or same-sex dormitory rooms.

- Linens and blankets (or sleeping bags and liners) will be provided.

- Towels are not part of the package. Take your own. Leave it behind if you won't be using it again at another YH. No need to carry the extra weight.

- You'll be sharing toilets and showers with others.

- There will probably be no place, other than your own pack, for locking up valuables (money, passport, credit/debit card). Although YHs are generally safe, you may wish to take valuables with you when you leave your dormitory room.

- Keep a flashlight handy for night excursions to the loo.

- Guests may be required to do KP after meals.

- Upon arrival you'll be asked to show your YH membership card, or to purchase one, which you can use at other hostels for a year. The card will make a nice souvenir bookmark when you return home.

- Check on the time your YH opens each evening. If possible, arrive then, so you can choose the room and bunk bed you prefer.

- You can, and we do, make reservations well in advance at Youth Hostels.

Black Sail Hut Youth Hostel

On the second night of our Coast to Coast Walk, we stayed in one of the most spartan and remote YHs in England. It loomed before me like a test of fortitude before I left home. A converted bothy (shepherd's shelter), Black Sail Hut once protected herdsmen from the wicked weather common in the Lake District. I knew in advance that this was a hostel with few amenities—no running water or electricity in its dormitories. What I didn't know was how grateful I would be to have stayed there.

Trail guides occasionally distort reality. Ours describes today's slog as a "scenic lakeside trail." And, I suppose, in clear weather Haweswater, and the hills that hug it, are a view to behold. The peaks that rise above the lake, however, have been obscured by rain that has been moistening us for hours.

During this hard, unpleasant day, I focus on my feet and the polished rocks beneath them, as I slip and slide atop slimy surfaces. I ford twenty-one brooks, becks, rills, and other water flows by jumping across or balancing on stones that protrude like the shells of submerged turtles. Often, my leaps fall short. My waterproofing is working overtime, but my good sportsmanship is growing soggy.

Eventually, we leave the lakeshore to follow a remote valley path. A few miles along, Mike spies a desolate black dot in the distance. "That must be it," I mutter from inside a dripping rain hood. "The end of fourteen wet miles of misery." The primitive structure emerging from the mist, however, is not reassuring.

Black Sail Hut Youth Hostel is a snug little building with a main room for eating and two attached dormitory rooms. Trudging from the common room to our sleeping quarters, the loo, or the one unheated shower (which I do not intend to use) requires venturing outside. This may be camping with amenities, but there are too few for me. I am wet and weary and whiny when Mike pushes open the door.

My first impression, as we duck under lines draped with the unmentionables of strangers, is that we have entered a tenement. Clothes drip from every surface. Boots dry perched atop ceiling beams. Sleeping bags hang from rafters. A stout wood stove looks lost beneath curtains of fabric.

We are the last to arrive and check in. Seven soggy guests observe our entrance in wary silence. Is my unhappiness that obvious as I view the situation? As I discover that there are no lines left for our wet things, that our bunks will be the leftovers no one else has claimed, that only one toilet is functioning, and that eleven of us will have to share the remaining outdoor, rustic facility?

"No, youth hostels do not provide towels," the innkeeper replies, when I request one to take to my unheated room.

"Well, I didn't know that, and I really need one," I reply. "I'm drenched and rapidly turning to ice." I'm also tired and growing ornery, but refrain from adding this.

"Sorry," says our tyrannical host, "If you didn't bring your own, I can't help you."

This exchange takes place in front of the other bedraggled strangers. What must they be thinking about this pushy American who hasn't read her YH rules in advance? I really don't care. Mike, however, is getting his "I don't know this woman" look.

"Okay, I'll take one of those," I say pointing to a dish towel in the kitchen behind her. "Used will be fine. Or maybe a few paper towels if that's all you have." Mike has retreated from the fray and is hiding behind a dripping slicker.

"Well," she says—the rock is budging—"Let me see if another guest has left one behind."

A fluffy towel appears. I'm set. But Mike is too mortified to prolong the scene by asking for one for himself. He just wants out.

The silence continues until I notice a guest with the power to lift even *my* spirits. A black and white terrier/greyhound mix is warming herself by the stove. Her tail thumps as I approach. In response to my hug, she treats me to a lovely lick. For the first time in hours, I relax.

"Do you like dogs?" asks a tall, strong woman about my age.

"No. We love dogs," I reply.

She smiles and relaxes with me. Margaret introduces herself, then explains that dogs are not allowed in youth hostels, but that her family group is rather stuck, miles from a B & B. If they can't stay here, there's no where else for them—or Poppy—to sleep. I understand. It's the reason we're here as well.

Miss Tyranny (who, it seems, has a heart after all) has agreed to allow Poppy's party of five to stay the night if none of the other guests objects to having her in residence. Margaret's family has been waiting for us, the final guests, to arrive, worrying about our verdict. Now, the jury is in. Poppy stays! The crisis passes, conversation picks up, and we begin settling in.

Settling in means finding a place between bunk beds in the ladies' dorm to store my damp pack. I notice the other women have been kind enough to leave some floor space and a windowsill near my bunk for me to unpack my things. I'll be sleeping on an upper bunk—presumably, the warmer bed, assuming heat rises—which means I'll probably disturb my three roommates when I climb down during the night to visit the loo. They tell me not to worry, that they sleep soundly. And they do.

Margaret and the others also clear some space for us to dry our clothes on a line in the main room. Mike and I are surprised that we have very few wet things to hang up. We used pack covers all day, and everything inside our packs was in plastic bags. Only our boots and socks, rain pants and jackets, pack covers and gaiters, and some sweaty underwear are on display in public. We are grateful not to be as soaked through as some of our companions.

Dinner is a vegetarian meal, shared at a long table, seasoned with tales from other treks. While washing up afterwards, we learn that there is a road to the YH that we could have walked easily, without the stones and streams that made our way so unpleasant. But that's okay. We're here now. And we're with friends—safe and dry and sleepy.

I wonder as I burrow into my comforter-like sleeping bag whether I'll be warm enough to sleep. But I don't wonder for long. Like bears in a den, we four "girls" produce enough calories to warm our tiny unheated cave, which soon becomes positively cozy.

In the morning, I'm feeling refreshed and ready to pamper my bunk-mates. Before they wake, I venture outside, dressed only in long under-wear, to take our common jug (pitcher) to the kitchen and negotiate with Miss Tyranny for some of the water she's heating on the stove. I carry it back to share with those who have welcomed and cared for me. "How lovely," they say. "How ever did you get warm water?" My answer is a smile.

By breakfast I'm getting the hang of this youth hosteling thing, al-most liking it. Maybe because it's nearly over. Maybe because it's forced me to leave my comfort zone and step away from the familiar into adven-ture and possibility. Maybe because the sun has come out to welcome us, and I'm grateful for this beautiful day.

After we wash our dishes, I return my towel and humbly thank our host for putting up with me. Seven of us leave together, scrambling up the very steep hill that marks our first half-mile. Poppy leads the way.

Soon we spread out, making plans to meet further down the Coast to Coast path. At the top of the hill, I look down at the black spot that sheltered us, the cocoon from which I emerged a better rambler. I throw it a kiss before turning and walking on.

Only 168 miles to go to Robin Hood's Bay and the end of the Coast to Coast Walk.

Note: We didn't know it then, but in the years to come we would enjoy many miles of walking on other paths that cross the English countryside with some of the friends we made at Black Sail Hut.

Step 8

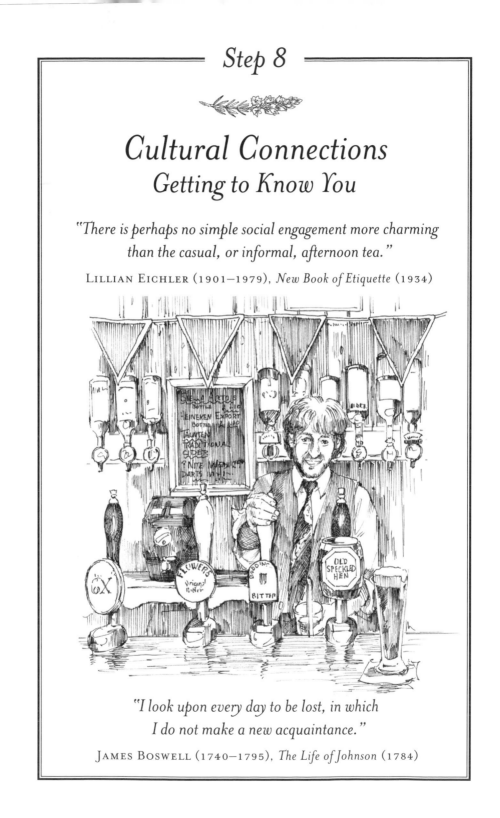

Cultural Connections
Getting to Know You

"There is perhaps no simple social engagement more charming than the casual, or informal, afternoon tea."

LILLIAN EICHLER (1901–1979), *New Book of Etiquette* (1934)

"I look upon every day to be lost, in which I do not make a new acquaintance."

JAMES BOSWELL (1740–1795), *The Life of Johnson* (1784)

Proper: The One and Only Way

Sustenance

The Joy of Guilt-Free Eating
Pub Pudding
A Pub for All Reasons
    TIP 8.1: Pub Survival
Full English Breakfast—Offa's Dyke Path
Lunch on the Go—Offa's Dyke Path
A Nice Cuppa
    TIP 8.2: Tea for You
Dinner Bell
    TIP 8.3: Dining Dos

Warm and Toasty

Fellow Ramblers

Cast of Characters—Coast to Coast Walk
    Roughing It
    Friends in Need
    Friends to the End
Reunions: Out and About Together
    Cotswold Outing
    Offa's Dyke Ramble

Hard to Say

English-Yankee Vocabulary
    TIP 8.4: Speaking "Proper" English on Holiday
A Way with Words

Proper: The One and Only Way

"Proper" is the gold standard in Great Britain. It's the seal of approval, an assurance that customs will be preserved as they are meant to be. And they are meant to be British.

Proper porridge is made with milk. Proper toast sits upright on a table in little metal cooling racks. Proper sandwiches are buttered. Proper English breakfasts require a day of walking to clear one's arteries. Proper footpaths build orienteering skills. And proper walking attire includes a plastic map case hanging about one's neck.

A proper B & B throws open its windows and doors to invite in fresh air in all seasons—weather conditions are irrelevant. Proper sinks have two taps, one for scalding, the other for chilling, and no device for mixing the two. The proper time for turning on heat at a B & B is between five and seven in the evening—after guests have had their baths and left for the pub—and again at seven in the morning—after walkers have already shivered into their clothing.

As far as I can tell, "proper" is authentic when it is either slightly uncomfortable or a bit inconvenient, and especially if it involves some suffering (hence, the hard toast and cold rooms). Proper builds stamina. It makes one's upper lip suitably stiff. It never coddles. It doesn't make exceptions. It's the standard to which both natives and visitors are held. It is rather quirky, often charming, and clearly British.

But don't worry. You needn't know its rules in advance. When the time is right—or even when it isn't—people will step forward to tell you what's proper. And when they do, don't bother to argue or negotiate. Second opinions don't count.

Sustenance

THE JOY OF GUILT-FREE EATING

I've been eating unbelievable amounts of food. Full meals and large portions, with candy bars in between. And my trousers still fit! Actually, they're a little loose. Shrinking hips are the "proof of the pudding" that countryside walking is a caloric big-burn.

When you're rambling, food tastes great. Every meal appeals, every dessert is "free food." You enter a privileged fantasy world of unrestrained dining where calories seem to vanish, and waistlines stay the course. Wear a pack, walk the miles, and you can forget about adding inches. It's enough to make one a vagabond.

Pub Pudding

I've consumed my vegetarian lasagna and mushy peas, and I'm still hungry, but not hesitant. I'm going for dessert, confident that, even after my filling pub lunch, the miles ahead will burn off an optional sweet. Calories have become irrelevant!

I march back to the bar, where we ordered our main course, to review the list of "puddings" ("desserts" in colonial-speak) posted on the wall. I select the third one down because I have no idea what it is. And nothing is as thrilling as a new dessert. Mustering my courage, I mumble, "For table three, please. One… spotted dick."

Heads turn. Silence falls. "Could you repeat that, mum?"

"Spotted dick," I blurt out a bit too loudly, expecting the patrons at the bar to snicker in amusement. But they do not. To my surprise they nod approvingly and return to their drinks. Apparently, I've made a "proper" selection after all!

The dessert challenge met, my dignity somewhat intact, I return with my prize to Mike (who, to this day, will not order his own spotted dick). My spongy cake square, freckled with currants, and covered in thick caramel sauce, promises to be a pudding well worth the teasing.

A Pub for All Reasons

No establishment is quite like the British pub. It is a favorite watering hole, a focus of village life, and an appealing antidote to fast-food sameness. Pubs are the "go-to" places where families eat, dogs and visitors mingle, and pints of naturally carbonated, regional ales are hand pumped from basement casks by bartenders with biceps. Pubs have charming names, mostly average (but sometimes excellent) food, and are now smoke-free. The local pub is one of the best features of countryside walking. It is here you'll exchange toasts and stories at the end of a satisfying day.

Many pubs offer bed and breakfast accommodations at reasonable rates. Should you book a room for the night, be sure to request a quiet one (not one located directly over the bar).

If you plan to have dinner at a local pub, ask your B & B host to book a reservation for you. Pubs—especially in season—are very popular with locals and walkers alike. A reservation will prevent you from suffering a bout of low blood-sugar impatience while waiting in the bar for a table.

Your B & B host may offer to drive you to and from dinner. Or she may suggest that you walk a short distance for your meal. Just be certain that the distance really is short before agreeing to go it alone. Bear in mind that when you're ravenous and tired, a mile seems a lot longer. And, by all means, if you're walking to dinner, carry a torch (flashlight). Speeding drivers will see you sooner. And your socks and sandals will stay cleaner if you spy cow, sheep, and dog deposits before you step in them.

Some pubs supply packed lunches; others will tempt you to stop along your path for lunch or a cool drink. A pub is a shelter in the rain, a loo in the wilderness, and a source of local information and gossip. Most open for dinner at 6:30 or 7:00 PM. And, as any hungry walker will tell you, just about every pub is worth the wait.

Tip : 8.1 Pub Survival

- Don't worry if at first you feel a bit awkward in a pub. Feeling awkward is normal for outsiders.

- Expect to be treated as a minor curiosity, a new face among familiar ones.

- Folks may want to chat with you. And you, most certainly, will want to talk with them.

- When you arrive, order drinks at the bar where you see the beer taps. Try the "real ale" local brews. These are exceptional almost everywhere and particularly good in Yorkshire. Mixed juices delivered in bottles are tasty as well.

- Read the daily "specials board" (usually located close to the bar) and then place your food order. Sometimes this must be done a few feet from where you placed your drink order. But you won't know this until you're asked to move several steps along the bar from where you're standing. Just do it. Don't try to make sense of it.

- Ask for a menu if the "specials board" does not appeal, and proceed to the proper spot for placing orders.

- When you order your meal, expect the regulars at the bar to quiet down. This makes it easy for everyone to hear and comment on what a visitor plans to eat.

- Local custom determines when and where you pay. Credit/debit cards are generally accepted.

- The cigarette haze of the past is no longer part of the pub scene. Since July 2007, pubs and other indoor, public places have been smoke-free.

- Sometimes you will be able to wait at a low table in the bar area for your meal. Don't attempt to cross your legs under the miniature table. Your legs won't cross. Most pub furniture was designed centuries ago for much shorter people, and it hasn't changed.

- Your name or number will be called when your meal is placed on your table in the dining area.

- Pudding (dessert) can be ordered from your waiter or by returning to the bar. Local custom prevails.

- Most pubs have espresso machines. Very few pubs offer brewed decaf coffee.

- If you pass an open pub during the day and wish to use its loo or WC—that is, its "facilities"—step inside, and ask if you may do so. I have never been turned away.

- If you are not carrying a cell phone rented or purchased in the UK (ones from home may not work), a pub is a convenient place for making phone calls. If you do not have an international calling card and need to use the public phone at the bar, expect the patrons to listen to your conversation, as they help you feed handfuls of coins into the phone while time runs down.

- Ask your B & B hosts to make a dinner reservation for you at the pub if they think you'll need one. Eat early. You'll be hungry.

- Remember that people know each other in a village. Don't complain about your B & B at the pub. Your host will have heard what you said before she prepares your breakfast!

- Some pubs pack lunches for walkers. If you want one, ask about this at dinner. In warm weather, ask the cook to omit chocolate treats. They will melt and make a mess.

- The local pub—familiar, cozy, and convenient—is a walker's home away from home. The pity is that too many of these welcoming friends are disappearing from village life. So enjoy them while you can.

FULL ENGLISH BREAKFAST — OFFA'S DYKE PATH

Sunshine fills Alison's restored, eighteenth century dining room, promising a fine day ahead. Delicate china graces the polished Georgian table. At each place setting is a grapefruit half. Beyond is a selection of homemade jams, Alison's special marmalades, and a jar of Marmite, a brown yeast extract spread that tastes a bit like a bullion cube, but appeals to the British savory palate.

The sideboard offers an array of "starters." We help ourselves to fruit compote, juice, yogurt, and cold cereals set in attractive canisters. Our choices include Weetabix (a form of shredded wheat), granola, corn flakes, bran flakes, and some sort of sugar-coated pellets.

Last night we placed our order for the hot course to follow, which for Mike and me begins with porridge (oatmeal) prepared, no doubt, with cream or milk. With this, Alison serves brown (whole wheat) toast, each piece set vertically into its own section of a metal holder to ensure that the slices will be crisp—but also cold and hard—when consumed. We have a choice of tea, coffee, or hot cocoa. We choose strong black tea, which we dilute with a bit of hot water from a dainty porcelain pot.

The main fare is next. Our British walking companion has requested a full English breakfast: a plate of eggs, sausages, and bacon, served with grilled tomatoes and mushrooms, to which Alison has added fried potatoes.

Mike and I, preferring to limit our cholesterol intake, avoid the meat and eggs. As quasi-vegetarians, we request a slightly different main course: toast covered with baked beans (a staple in British homes) and an order of grilled mushrooms and tomatoes. Our choice is plenty filling after the fruit, toast, oatmeal, and yogurt.

As we bid Alison, her husband, their dog, and their lovely home adieu, we wonder how far we'll have to waddle before we feel spry enough to walk normally again.

Lunch on the Go—Offa's Dyke Path

At breakfast we ask if we might have some extra toast on which to spread homemade condiments to make sandwiches for lunch. Our host offers us some fruit to add to our fare (and our pack weight). Mike and I fold our marmalade sandwiches into a paper breakfast napkin and return to our room where we slip our treats into a spare plastic bag. Robin chooses to fill his sandwich with his uneaten sausage and egg from breakfast.

On other walks, we have enjoyed leisurely picnics under way, consuming generous lunches packed by B & B hosts. But Robin, an experienced rambler, prefers small, frequent snacks. So, on this journey we've been trying his style of eating. For the past one hundred miles, it's been working well.

In addition to our breakfast sandwiches and fruit, we carry energy bars and candy bars. Robin also has a stash of butterscotch hard candies, and I am lugging a package of artery-clogging Scottish shortbread—a treat well worth the extra weight and cardiac risk.

Two hours out, when we stop for biological necessities, we consume our first snack. At other stops, we eat other treats. Living off our reserves from breakfast, stoking our furnaces with calories throughout the day, we have plenty of energy to go the distance to our next B & B without lapsing into a hypoglycemic fog as the miles pass underfoot.

A Nice Cuppa

On the penultimate evening of our fifth walk, a two-hundred-mile journey along the Offa's Dyke Path, we stop in Bodfari at a B & B where tea is served with flare. Mrs. E greets us with a smile, offers a firm handshake, and leads us to a table in her garden. Minutes later, she places before us a stack of homemade Welsh tea cakes, a bowl of homegrown plums, and a pot of tea, along with milk, sugar, and some extra hot water. Robin asks for coffee, as he always does. (So much for tradition.) His coffee is served, as it is in most restaurants, pubs, and homes, in a French press.

Relaxed, my muscles at rest, sock-covered toes wiggling at will, I gaze south over the miles we have covered and the steep hills we have climbed. I'm filled with pleasure, contentment, gratitude, and Welsh tea cakes. With just one more day to Prestatyn and the end of our journey, we add Bodfari to other special tea moments tucked into our pack of memories.

Our seventh day out along the South Downs Way ends with a similarly memorable teatime experience. At our B & B in Amberly, we join Mrs. J in her kitchen, which is filled with late afternoon light. We are treated to homemade lemon layer cake and conversation about dog behavior, local doings, and Mrs. J's memories of World War II. We return to our room revived and refreshed, pleased that our tea for three has turned strangers into friends.

I also recall cozy afternoons in B & B bedrooms, heating water in white, plastic, electric kettles. This is the norm in homes with busy hosts and no common space for socializing. Some hosts leave candy bars to sweeten the solitary fare. Others provide biscuits. A few offer nothing. By late afternoon, out of energy and devoid of inhibition, I may ask if there are any biscuits in the kitchen. If not, "toast and jam will do." Only one host in over nine hundred miles of walking said, "No. Very sorry. You'll soon be having your dinner at the pub, won't you?" Fortunately, such unpleasantness is the exception, and generosity is the rule.

Teatime on a walk, like sharing a pint of ale at a local pub, is an invitation to rest, reflect, and celebrate a job well done. It is a perfectly lovely excuse to unwind and indulge. So take a few moments, and relax with a "nice cuppa," be it tea or coffee.

TIP : 8.2 TEA FOR YOU

  - A "nice cuppa" is a perfect reward at the end of any day.

  - Teatime will refresh and invigorate. So pause each day to enjoy this civilized national ritual in the company of others or in the quiet of your own room. Unpacking and bathing will wait.

  - Before having your tea, change into dry clothing to avoid a chill.

- Pubs normally serve dinner about 7 PM, and you may have several hours to wait after tea until you eat. Don't be afraid to ask for biscuits (cookies) or a sweet (candy) if these are not offered, your private cache of snacks is dwindling, and your blood-sugar is low. You can ask for toast and jam if all else fails.
- If you prefer, have coffee or cocoa instead of tea.

DINNER BELL

Yes, Virginia, there is fine food in Britain. If you're not a vegetarian, I have one culinary thing to say: Think lamb. Especially if you're in the Yorkshire Dales or Cumbria. And absolutely, if the lamb featured is of the Herdwick breed, found most commonly in the Lake District.

Meals in pubs and restaurants vary greatly, but fresh, local leg of lamb is almost always good, especially in the autumn. And where food is good, a reservation is advised. Since there are so few places to dine in many villages, it's normally a good idea to ask your host when you book your room (as noted earlier in this chapter and in Step Four) to make a dinner reservation for you for the evening you'll be staying with her. Hungry walkers are happier when they hold a reservation and dine at, or near, a restaurant's opening time.

If you're a vegetarian, be assured: England is friendly territory. You will almost always find something palatable on the menu. If nothing appeals, you have three fallback positions. First, helpings of steamed veggies are served as part of most meals, so you can request plain pasta or rice and steamed vegetables. Second, there may be an Indian or Chinese restaurant close by. And third, if all else fails, order the ubiquitous jacket potato—a large baked spud topped with almost anything you request: cole slaw, tuna salad, broccoli and cheese, baked beans, and more. Delicious.

The best and most convenient place to have dinner, however, is at your own B & B. If an evening meal is available, request it when you make your reservation. You will not be disappointed. Every B & B host has a few fine meals in his or her repertoire. And since you'll be staying only one night, your host will probably serve one of these. All of our in-home meals have been excellent—except for those that have been outstanding.

When booking your room and an evening meal, tell your host/chef your eating preferences and prohibitions. (See "Confirming Reservations" in Step Four.) You may wish to request lamb or fish or some other specialty. Hosts really try to do their best for you. A few may dine with you. Most will serve you and disappear. But all will be happy to have you dining in their homes. And no one will be happier than you when you do so.

TIP : 8.3 DINING DOS

· If you can, make reservations for dining out.

· If you're not a vegetarian, think lamb.

· If you prefer vegetarian fare, plenty of choices are available.

· When you can, arrange to have an evening meal at your B & B.

· British food—even pub food—is underrated. It is certainly more appetizing and interesting than most American fast food.

· Be assured: After a day of walking, almost all food tastes like fine cuisine.

Warm and Toasty

If you are never cold, Britain is the place for you. Energy is expensive and used sparingly. Homes are under-heated and over-ventilated. Fresh air flows in through open doors and swishes out through open windows, regardless of outdoor temperatures.

Heat may be available during certain, well-defined hours, but only if a house is cold enough and the weather nasty enough to meet British standards. Kitchens are almost always comfortable, but walkers are seldom invited to congregate with the family close to the kitchen stove. Space heaters may be available, but you'll probably have to ask (make that "beg") for one.

The cost of a kilowatt-hour doesn't fully account for this national aversion to warmth. It does not explain, for example, why discomfort has become a test of character, why low indoor temperatures invite smugness, or why the proper response to shivering should be stoicism.

One does, of course, adapt. I carry a selection of warm clothing to layer on as needed. And there's good news: Even cursed as I am with an American thermostat, I'm never cold while walking. Nor do I need extra layers once I'm tucked into bed under a plush British duvet. Stumbling along an unheated corridor to a cold bathroom at night, however, is another matter.

I gained some insight into how unsuitable my thermostat is for the great British indoors by observing Robin, our native walking companion. More than well-adapted, he's a living example of "snug as a bug."

Sitting across the table from me during our evening meal at a B & B, Robin is dressed for a summer barbecue. Having removed the light fleece jacket in which he arrived, he is sitting comfortably in a short sleeve golf shirt. At least he's wearing trousers rather than shorts. So I'm not completely demoralized, dressed, as I am, in my long sleeve, zip-tee underwear top and a nylon shirt, over which I've layered a fleece vest. My three-hundred-weight fleece jacket hangs on the back of my chair, and I am thinking about putting it on.

Robin has been training for this comfort contest for decades. He grew up without central heating. As an undergraduate at Cambridge, he lived in an unheated room and suffered cold showers. Chilly British Air Force assignments further honed his cold tolerance. I know I'm dining with a pro, and I'm impressed.

Adapting to chilly temperatures starts early in British life. Dressed in four fleecy layers, waiting for a train on a brisk fall day in Winchester at the end of our South Downs Way walk, I notice a mother in a light jacket seated on a nearby bench. She has a busy five-year-old in tow, who is dressed in shorts and a short sleeve shirt. He is well-mannered, but quite active. He seems to be having difficulty settling down in temperatures that hover around the fifty degree mark. Finally, I hear him tell his mum, "It's cold today, isn't it?"

Patting his adorable blonde head, but not reaching into her shopping bag for the sweater I'm certain will appear, she replies calmly, "Yes, it is." That's it. That's all she says. And not a peep do I hear from the little fellow, who seems destined for a chilly, but happy, future, dressed in short sleeve golf shirts.

Strange as it seems, I'm well acquainted with "serious cold," living as I do twenty minutes south of the Canadian border, where we consider warmth a friend worth inviting into our lives. We haul and stack wood for wood stoves. We install block heaters in car engines. We have double-paned glass in our windows and double thick insulation in our walls. We go to a lot of trouble and expense keeping the cold outdoors where it belongs.

This is why I'm not defensive about my preference for warmth, even when confronting an ardent B & B host, who asserts that a room heated above sixty degrees will break down my immune system and cause dehydration.

First, I explain that I'm willing to take those risks. Then I ask for a little more heat.

Fellow Ramblers

Some of the people whom we have met on our journeys have become fast friends with whom we continue to correspond and share new adventures.

Paul Millmore is, perhaps, the person most responsible for introducing us to countryside walking. Mike met Paul, who is the author of the *South Downs Way*—National Trail Guide, while on vacation in England. Paul encouraged us to give walking in Britain a try, promising it would be relaxed, comfortable, and dramatically different from hiking the peaks in New York State's Adirondack Park, which is less than an hour from our home. With some trepidation, we decided to do as he suggested. In fact, we launched our first walk from his home, happy to have his family's good wishes and sound advice.

And it was to his home that we returned at the end of the South Downs Way to celebrate with his family the completion of our first ramble—and to report that we were totally hooked.

CAST OF CHARACTERS — COAST TO COAST WALK

We met several other walking friends on our third ramble, the Coast to Coast Walk across England. This two-hundred-mile path from St. Bees on the Irish Sea to Robin Hood's Bay on the North Sea promotes bonding. If you meet a stranger, you walk together. If you need directions, someone will stop to show you the way. If you book into a B & B with other ramblers, you'll chat over tea and meet later at the pub for a meal. Faces grow familiar, and friendships deepen.

Roughing It

We met a family group in the Lake District at Black Sail Hut Youth Hostel after a wet day our second night out: Mike F and his wife, Margaret; Colin, Margaret's brother; and Colin's eighteen-year-old daughter, Frances. (See Step Seven, "Black Sail Hut Youth Hostel" for details.) Our shared experience of soggy clothing and a night of basic living drew us together. Poppy, their enthusiastic, greyhound-terrier mix, sealed the relationship. We shared two additional evening meals before they left us half-way along the Coast to Coast path to return home. They planned to return the following year to complete their final one hundred miles—which, I am pleased to report, they did.

Friends in Need

We met David and Sheila on a steep slope outside Grasmere, where we helped each other locate the route to follow. We met again during lunch overlooking Grisdale Tarn. Still later, in Orton, when we found ourselves staying at the same local hotel, we joined them for dinner. David and Sheila, who were using a luggage carrying service, remarked on the pack I was carrying, but did not ask why I needed to carry so much. Instead, Sheila said that she admired my strength and stamina, which was the perfect thing to say to a mildly defensive "what-if" walker. No wonder we became friends.

We were to cement our friendship several days later when we met at the end of a truly awful day climbing over Nine Standards Rigg in the rain, wind, and fog. Mike and I hobbled for miles on weary ankles, perching ourselves atop tufts of grass, leaping across streams, trying to avoid the waist-deep muck of the upland bog that mired other walkers and blackened their rain gear.

With this dreadful trek behind us, and still managing to stay upright on tired and unsteady legs, we arrived at a phone booth in the late afternoon. I had walked enough for one day. I shivered while Mike called a taxi to take us two miles into Thwaite to our inn for the night.

David and Sheila emerged from the mist a few minutes later. I will be forever indebted to Sheila for looking as cold and as miserable as I felt and for whining and complaining with me. At times like these "misery loves company," and "stiff upper lip" would be totally out of place. Four of us shared the taxi.

Friends to the End
Taking a day off in Richmond introduced us to a new group of coast-to-coasters, who had been walking a day behind us. At Danby Wiske, the first night after our day of rest, the couple who would be sharing our bathroom arrived at our B & B in time to have tea with us. That evening we joined Robin and Joan for the worst pub meal any of us has ever suffered. Microwaved, prepackaged everything, smothered in gooey cheese, became the glue of a new friendship.

We walked together, sharing several pleasant days and decent meals before Robin and Joan rambled on ahead, following an itinerary more ambitious than ours. They finished one day ahead of us, which we confirmed at Robin Hood's Bay in the traditional way of Coast to Coast walkers who succeed in reaching this hard-won destination.

We enter the pub overlooking the North Sea, order two half-pints, and ask for "the book." We are handed a bound, black volume that looks like a ship's log. Opening it, we scan the names. There they are. David and Sheila. Robin and Joan. We've done it! All of us!

Pen in hand, we place our names and thoughts below theirs: "18 September 1998," we write. "We did it all and have arrived at last whole and happy." Toasting our success, we linger over our ales—but not too long. Another tradition awaits.

Just outside, the North Sea is lapping at the cobblestones where the pavement ends. Marching to the water's edge to mark our accomplishment, we dip our boots into the sea, the same boots that stepped into the Irish Sea almost three weeks ago on the morning our journey began.

REUNIONS: OUT AND ABOUT TOGETHER
Cotswold Outing
On a sunny day, two years after our Coast to Coast walk, Colin, Margaret, Mike F, and Poppy join us and Robin and Joan for a day of walking on the

Cotswold Way. As we move down the path together, pleasantly accented chatter fills my ears and feeds my spirit.

Drawn together by our C-to-C experiences, our new friends have left jobs and obligations and driven several hours to walk with us again. They will be spending two nights away from home, either caravan camping or checked into our B & Bs. We are dazzled by their warmth and kindness and inspired by their example. We resolve to follow their lead and make time to visit with other friends when we return home.

A few hours into our walk, we leave the trail to rest at a pub, which Margaret, a seasoned map reader, has located off-trail for us. After hydrating and using the facilities, I return to my pack and prepare to put it on. The five natives, transformed now into a band of rambling friends, ask me if I am planning to walk on without them.

"Well," I say, "I am thinking we'd best be on our way. We have about ten miles ahead of us, and it's nearly noon."

"But we're about to order lunch," Mike F says. "And then we have to eat it. So why don't you put down your pack, and decide what you want."

The band is in agreement. Today's pace will be leisurely, with time for fun and friendship. Distance doesn't concern them. Finishing in fading daylight doesn't trouble them.

I want to remember this lesson as life at home speeds up. When miles of commitments stretch before me and I start to worry about going the distance, I want to remember that I have a choice and that I can choose to travel at a more leisurely pace.

Offa's Dyke Ramble

Several years later some of us gather to step out again. This time, Mike and I have selected the Offa's Dyke Path, and Robin has decided to join us, making our journey a nineteen-day reunion. Although Joan is busy and cannot walk with us, she is as near as Robin's cell phone, but not, unfortunately, near enough for "girl talk" en route.

Happily, Margaret and Mike F, along with irrepressible Poppy, walk the first three (shakedown) days with us, camping in their caravan each evening. Twelve days later David and Sheila arrive in a remote village to join Mike, Robin, and me for a day of motoring in the Welsh countryside. (See Step Four, "Full Day to Explore.")

For most of the time on the Offa's Dyke path, however, it is just the three of us. Robin, our unofficial guide and interpreter of all things English, wears a plastic map case around his neck and keeps his GPS at the ready. Uncomplaining, always patient, he hides the map from me whenever its topographic lines converge into what look like bundles of fiber optic cable, a sign that serious up-or-downhill effort lies ahead.

Mike, our naturalist and navigational consultant, stops for birds and planes overhead, both of which he and Robin feel compelled to identify. He supports Robin in map cover-ups, unless I swear to resist topo panic.

"All I want is a peek at the book," I tell them.

"No need," says Mike. "Nothing here to worry about."

"A piece of cake," says Robin.

I don't believe them, of course. But, by now, this is a game we all agree to enjoy.

My niche is "official stile counter," slowpoke, and supervisor of rest stops and photo-ops. When I stop, everyone stops.

In nineteen days on the Offa's Dyke Path, trekking over two hundred miles, ascending 23,000 feet of accrued elevation and climbing over some 488 stiles, we never run out of stories. We never tire of seeing the patchwork landscape of green countryside. We never pass a walker without a conversation. We never remember all the lyrics to the songs we sing.

Eventually, I stop worrying about the hills I have to climb. Robin and Mike can identify most of the birds we see. And then it's over. How did so many days disappear? Where will we go on our next walk? How soon will we be together again?

Hard to Say

When we first learn our mother tongue, we have to decipher its words, put them into context, and master hundreds of new expressions. This is what we still must do in foreign lands, even in places where people profess to speak our language—places like Australia, India, New Zealand, and, yes, Great Britain.

Accents are the first hurdle. In Scotland, Ireland, Yorkshire, and certain neighborhoods in London, Manchester, and Liverpool, spoken

English may require translation. In Wales, where travelers find the native tongue indecipherable, folks also speak English, but you may have to work to understand them.

To local accents, add local expressions, and you'll know you're not in Kansas anymore. For example, to the question, "Can you tell me where our laundry is drying," you may receive an answer, phrased as a question, which sounds like a reprimand: "Your laundry is in the drying closet, isn't it." Or, "I've pegged it on the line outside, haven't I." Be assured—those final words are added to express certainty, aren't they. They are not put-downs tacked on to insult you.

Other sentences end with a little stab for emphasis, in the form of the words "this" or "that." It's the British equivalent of "n'est-ce pas" (French), "Eh" (Canadian), and "Is it," "Isn't it," and "Ain't it" (American). You hear it in expressions like, "A very soft pillow, this," and "Not getting any better, that." Add a few "thises" and "thats" to your own sentences, and you'll be hooked.

Implied verbs are commonly expressed in the UK. Asked, for example, if I would book the same B & B again, I might reply, "Yes," or "I would." Robin, however, would reply, "Yes, I would do." And to my question, "Do you think we should have turned at that waymark fifteen minutes back?" Robin would, and, unfortunately did, reply, "Yes I think we should have done."

The English also shorten verbs. To my request, "Would you hand that teapot to me?" I was told, "Could do," meaning, "Right. I could do that for you." Also in vogue are "should do" and "would do," but not the American "can do."

Another difference in our "common language" is the use of the plural for collective nouns, as in "The team are playing their rival today," Or "The insurance company aren't going to like this." Or "Parliament are meeting now on that issue." Coming from the colonies, however, gives you a pass on "proper" subject-verb agreement, just as it does on the use of articles, which in England are occasionally dropped, as in, he's "in hospital," or, preferably, "on holiday."

Even simple words, however, may confuse the traveler when they mean one thing in American English and another in British English. For example, Brits "sort" things out while we "work" them out or "figure" them out. Brits are "keen" to do things that we merely "want" to do. For them, "brilliant" affirms the acceptable. It does not imply that your last utterance was fabulously insightful. In fact, the word often follows a mundane statement, such as, "Nancy says she'll be joining us for dinner." To which the proper reply is, "Brilliant."

ENGLISH-YANKEE VOCABULARY

· Transportation

bonnet = car hood

boot = car trunk

caravan = mobile home or recreational trailer

coach = bus

dual carriageway = divided highway

lorry = truck

metalled road = paved road

motorway = highway, freeway

roundabout = traffic circle

· Foods and Beverages

banger = sausage

biscuit = cookie or cracker

bitter = term for a well-hopped ale, normally on draft

chips = French fried potatoes

crisps = potato chips

granary bap = whole grain bread roll

jam = jelly (not preserves)

jelly = jello

jug = pitcher (Ask for a "jug" of water.)

pudding = desserts of all kinds, not just custards

sweet = candy

· Walking Terms

capel = chapel (Wales)

carreg = stone (Wales)

close – entrance

coomb (cwm in Wales) = narrow valley

dale = valley

downs = rolling uplands, usually grass-covered and without trees

glen = valley (Scotland)

fell = hill or mountain

moor = high, open area, often covered with heather or with peat bogs

pike = peak (Yorkshire)

public right-of-way = path or track open to the public

rigg = ridge

rucksack = backpack

tarn = small upland lake

trainers = sneakers

thwaite = clearing or meadow

verge = shoulder of a road

- **General**

anyroad = anyway (used in northern England, particularly in Yorkshire)

at the minute = at the moment

fag = cigarette

fagged = tired

flannel = washcloth

inn = a pub with overnight accommodations

jumper = sweater

pavement = sidewalk

rubber = eraser

scheme = a plan (not some nefarious plot)

torch = flashlight

TIP : 8.4 SPEAKING "PROPER" ENGLISH ON HOLIDAY

· Have fun trying out and brushing up your Brit-English before leaving home. Tune into British programs on public television. Use a "flannel" for bathing. And if you're chilly, reach for your "jumper."

- When necessary, ask locals to speak slowly, especially in Scotland and Yorkshire, where English can sound like a foreign language.

- Expect what you say and how you pronounce it to amuse your listeners. Certainly, their expressions will amuse you. "Garage," along with "barrage" and "Saint Bernard," sound as strange to the English when we accent the final syllable as the words sound to us with the accent on the first syllable.

- Be brave. Speak up. And enjoy our uncommon language.

A WAY WITH WORDS

For me, place names are the essence of British English. Colorful, descriptive, and original, they put American "white bread" proper nouns to shame. Compare our Smithtown or Niceville with their Chipping Campden and Waterley Bottom, our Ellenburg with their Kettlewell, or our Margaret Street with their Puck Pitt Lane.

Pubs, too, sport catchy, often obtuse, names exhibited on elaborate signs that beckon and tantalize the passerby. Who wouldn't want to drop by for a pint of bitter or a cappuccino at the White Hart Inn, Fox and Hound, Golden Fleece, Black Horse, King's Head, Dog Pub, or the fictional Drovers Arms of James Herriot fame.

My favorite British names, however, are those attached to houses and B & Bs. Displayed on signs that welcome the visitor, they are charming and creative. Some of my favorites include Hag's End (the farm so named was a near wreck), First Hurdle Guest House (our first stop on the Offa's Dyke Path), Rest for the Tired, Woodwinds, The Old Bakehouse, The Old Court House, Greencroft, Tarnclose, and The Rectory (a real rectory on the Ridgeway Path with a real rector as its host).

Home owners put out clever warning signs as well—many to encourage drivers to slow down. For example, one sign we passed read: "Free ranging children. Please drive slowly." Another warned: "Children playing with catapults and sharp sticks. Please drive slowly. Their aim is a bit off."

Signs are also directed at dog owners—a passionate and ubiquitous segment of a population that includes its dogs on rambles, invites canines into pubs, and travels with them on trains and coaches. This hand-painted gem was posted on a footpath where it crossed private property:

Be ye dog, or be ye bitch,
We love you all no matter which.
Respect our grass; respect it do.
And find elsewhere to do your pooh.

Brilliant!

Step 9

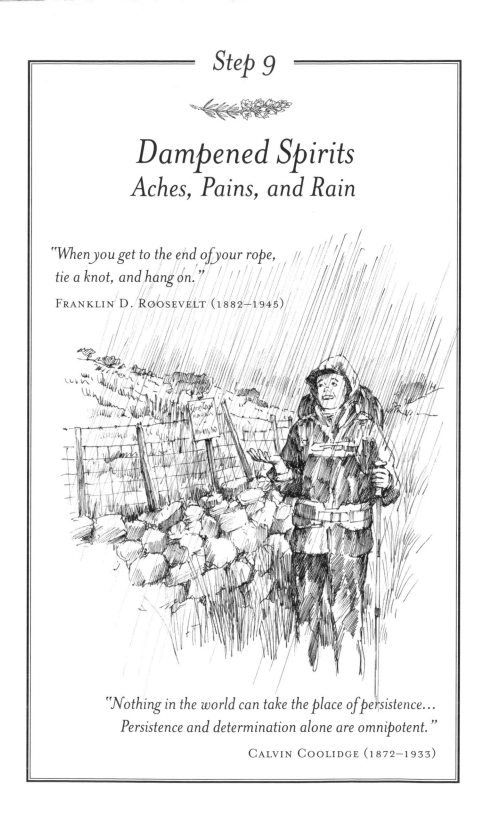

Dampened Spirits
Aches, Pains, and Rain

*"When you get to the end of your rope,
tie a knot, and hang on."*

FRANKLIN D. ROOSEVELT (1882–1945)

*"Nothing in the world can take the place of persistence...
Persistence and determination alone are omnipotent."*

CALVIN COOLIDGE (1872–1933)

Aches and Pains

JOURNAL: Ouch

Hobbling Along

JOURNAL: Dales Way Dilemna

TIP 9.1: Weaning Off Worry

JOURNAL: Offa's Dyke Backache

South Downs Way Blister - Mike's Turn

JOURNAL: Affliction

Blister Busters

TIP 9.2: Prevention Is Still the Best Treatment

Rainy Reflections

JOURNAL: Drenched

Dales Way Deluge

Keeping It Dry

TIP 9.3: Try for Dry

Rain (A Poem)

Attitude Adjustment

JOURNAL: Greetings

Pet Therapy

TIP 9.4: Canine Comforts

Grumpies

JOURNAL: I've Had It

TIP 9.5: Rx for Whiny Moments

Mid-Soul

JOURNAL: Halfway

Competitive Walking

Your Way Is Okay

TIP 9.6: What's Right for You Is Right

Special Places

JOURNAL: Stewards of the Land

Aches and Pains

> ## Ouch
>
> *I'm worried about a painful ankle. Will it hold up tomorrow when I put
> on my pack and we start our walk? Should I walk on it at all? Will it get
> worse if I favor it? Should I loosen my laces to relieve pressure, or does my
> ankle need support? I don't know what to do.* 🞰

HOBBLING ALONG

Three days ago, I thought our walk was over. We set out for a warm-
up ramble from Ilkley, where we were staying for two nights after our
overseas flight. Leaving our regular packs at the hotel, we gathered a few
things into a small day pack and walked to the neighboring village of
Addingham. It was from here that Mike's ancestors abandoned their lives
as weavers in the woolen trade and set sail for colonial America. We were
hopeful that local church records might provide information about his
relatives and the families they left behind.

But on the day we walked to Addingham the church office was locked,
its records unavailable. The date was 06 September 1997, the day of Princess Diana's funeral, a time of national sadness. Both Ilkley and Addingham were silent except for the chatter escaping through open windows
from tellies covering the event. Shops and pubs were closed until noon.
Pictures of a beautiful princess stared at us from impromptu shrines on
lawns and windowsills, in parks and storefronts.

We entered the churchyard in Addingham, hopeful that its barely
legible headstones might add a few details to Mike's family's story. I had
passed four graves when I came upon a stone with the crumbling names
we were seeking. "Over here," I called. "It's John and Mary! And others,
too."

Kneeling down I began reading the weathered markers. Here were
Mike's forebears—generations of them.

How long I remained in that posture, recording the births and deaths
of people I wish I had known, I can't remember. But when I straightened

up, I was certain our walk had ended before it had officially begun. In crouching down to read the stones, I injured my ankle. I stood up in serious pain.

Now, three days later, my ankle still hurts—a great deal—and I don't know what to do about it.

I've been moving forward on it, hoping that walking will not make it worse. It's still a bit swollen and sensitive to touch, but, thankfully, it's less painful than it was in the graveyard—even burdened, as it is now, by the added weight of my pack. Still, I worry. Will it hold up? Will I make it to the end of the trail? Should I be walking on it at all?

I ask Mike to refrain from asking about my injury. His concern—sweet as it is—triggers my own. Dwelling on—talking about—a problem that I can't do much about is upsetting. Better to focus on other things, like stone walls, stiles, and appealing villages. Better to avoid obsessing. Better to play the role of "positive person" and carry on.

My journal over several painful days, however, reveals that on a path paved with good intentions, good sportsmanship can get trampled.

❧ Journal

Dales Way Dilemna

Giving it a Try—Warm-up
Four Miles: Addingham to Base Camp in Ilkley

I only glance at the villages below our ridge-top trail. I'm not interested in talking about Mike's family history. I'm busy worrying about tomorrow and the twelve miles I'll have to walk on a bad ankle, carrying a twenty-three-pound pack. If I knew what was wrong with my ankle—sprain, strain, tear, chipped bone—I might figure out how to take care of it or choose to alter our plans. Or maybe I wouldn't. Maybe I'd just take a risk, move forward on it, and hope for the best—which is what I'm doing.

A little good news…heading back to Ilkley, I progressed from limping to almost painless walking. Uphill felt better than level. Level felt better than downhill. I almost look forward to trekking up hills. Still, I'm scared and feel very sorry for myself. I don't like being tested in this way.

I Think I Can—Day One
Twelve Miles: Ilkley to Howgill

My ankle is holding. Sometimes it's painful. Other times it's okay. Happily, it's less swollen today. I've decided to walk on it as long as I can. I'm not as worried as I was yesterday. On today's river walk, we viewed the skeletal grandeur of Bolton Abbey, which diverted my attention from my own discomfort to the misery created by King Henry VIII's ambition.

Over the Hump—Day Two
Six Miles: Howgill to Grassington

My ankle is not getting worse. It looks like I'll be able to live with it for another seventy miles. Since worrying about aches and pains seems to magnify them, I've been trying to forsake my fretful ways by ignoring my ankle and smiling a lot.

In the village of Grassington, on this short day of walking, we have time for a leisurely lunch (that includes a very chocolate cake for me) and a stroll along cobbled streets.

Although my stride is choppy, my ankle threatening, a blister starting, and unpleasant weather is in the forecast, I enjoy the lovely afternoon. I'll address other troubles if and when they occur.

I'm growing brave. I can visualize finishing. I'm beginning to feel like a rambler. 🪶

Postscript

We managed to complete the Dales Way and reach Bowness on Lake Windermere without detour or delay. After several months at home and with a doctor's diagnosis (a probable compressed nerve) to put my mind at ease, my ankle finally stopped hurting.

My one regret is not that I squatted in hiking boots to read aged gravestones. It's that I squandered too many happy moments on the trail worrying about something I couldn't change.

9.1 Weaning Off Worry

· It's okay to worry, just not too often. Fretting can become a habit.

· Save your worry for important things that require attention, like getting to the airport on time for your flight home.

· If you can't fix or mitigate a problem, limit the time you allow yourself to obsess about it.

· Write about what worries you, talk about what worries you, then focus on things that please you and make you smile.

· Worry, unchecked, diminishes pleasure and steals joy. It isn't worth the sacrifice.

❦ Journal

Offa's Dyke Backache

Scaling a ladder stile—and being reasonably careful and focused while doing so—I feel a sharp pain in my back. I'm afraid I've injured a disc. I've had experience with this malady, and I'm praying that the pain is merely a pulled muscle that will respond to a nonprescription pain reliever. Downhill I ache. Uphill I hurt. And tomorrow we face hundreds of feet of up hill and down dale.

Oddly, I feel more determined than worried, more frustrated than afraid. On the verge of tears, I'm angry that this is happening three nights and thirty-eight miles from Prestatyn at the end of the path. I've come so far. One hundred sixty-five glorious miles. I want to finish. 🦋

Postscript

I do finish, as planned. And three days later when we reach Prestatyn, I am feeling much better.

I'm not a driven, Olympic-type athlete. Yet, after hundreds of miles of walking, when pain strikes, my usual approach is to take care of it if I can and get through it if I must. I rarely think about giving in or giving up before reaching the end of a path.

From my core, a small voice propels me forward, whispering, "Take a risk. You'll be all right. Stop worrying. It's probably nothing. Walking is good for you." And, my favorite prompt: "You'll live."

So, assuming I can keep going, I carry on, *stepping out* toward the next mile marker, in the direction I'm meant to travel.

South Down's Way Blister—Mike's Turn

Journal

Affliction

Only the second day of our first British ramble, and Mike is suffering with a blister that covers the bottom of his foot just behind his toes. We can't wrap it, puncture it, or treat it in any way we know. It's almost all we talk about. We're afraid it will force us to cancel the rest of our walk. ✄

How, we ask ourselves, as Mike hobbles next to me on what might have been a lovely day, did this happen to us? Our answers make us feel guilty. We should have known better.

- We were too excited to fully appreciate the impact of the hard chalk surface hidden beneath the green downs carpet under our feet, as we pranced over the undulating Seven Sisters (seaside hills often mistaken for their more famous cousins, the White Cliffs of Dover). We proceeded inland and continued on to Alfriston. Distracted by the countryside and entranced by perfect weather, Mike ignored a minor discomfort at the bottom of his foot.
- We didn't stop often enough or long enough for him to air, cool, and dry his foot after it started to feel tender.
- Mike's boots were too wide for his ultra-narrow feet, even with his laces tied tight. His foot moved a bit inside his boot as we trekked the coastal hills—in spite of sock liners and heavy hiking socks. And friction creates blisters.
- Because of the added weight of his pack, he needed boot insoles with more cushioning to prevent wear and tear on his aging foot pads.
- We could have stopped for a day before the blister grew, so he could have iced and rested his foot. But we didn't. So now, what do we do?

We decide to take a day off, hoping that twenty-four hours of ice and rest will improve his condition and that we'll be able to complete the South Downs Way. We rebook our reservations and rest.

Postscript

Rested and in less pain, but still hobbling, Mike managed to carry on, feeling better each day as his blister metamorphosed into a callous. Nine days after we set out from Eastbourne, we arrived in Winchester at the end of the path, whole and happy.

Blister Busters

For generations, people have trod paths on feet just like ours, wearing ill-fitting, unforgiving footwear. Today, we have technical hiking boots, and yet we suffer as they did from a malady as old as the ages: blisters.

There are probably as many treatments for these burning bubbles as there are reasons for getting them. Every walker swears by some pet cure as *the* proven method for coping with them. Some cures work better than others. Below are several personal favorites of walkers who have fought the blister battles and claim to have won.

• If ice is available at your B & B, place it on tired, raw spots that could cause trouble before they do cause trouble.
• My own favorite blister buster is Dr. Scholl's® 100% Lamb's Wool Padding. As soon as I feel a blister coming on, I wrap a little bit of wool snugly around my sore toe. The wool felts to itself (and sometimes to my sock liner), but it stays in place. Each morning I rewrap the toe in question. Overlapping or troublesome toes should be wrapped in advance to prevent problems.
• Although many people prefer moleskin, Cathy (sixty-plus-years-old) swears by Dr. Scholl's® Cushlin™ Ultra Slim Blister Treatment for wilderness hiking. She also uses New-Skin® Liquid Bandage. Armed with these two remedies, Cathy traveled two hundred miles, carrying a thirty-five pound pack, on the Long Trail in Vermont. (What a girl!)
• Bob prefers Band-Aid® Blister Block, although he cautions that it has to be applied correctly in order to work. It can be placed on a fully

formed blister or used preventively. After covering an area, he leaves the Block on until a "second skin" forms. Then he removes it, taking care not to pull off the new skin beneath. This worked well for him for two hundred miles along the Thames Path.

- Robert and Elizabeth, married British physicians whom we met near the end of our Coast to Coast walk, told us that their favorite blister buster is in their sewing kit. They sterilize a needle, thread it with clean thread, and pass it through a blister, leaving the string behind. The blister, kept open by the string, slowly drains. This method is not for the squeamish, but it does seem to work. (Don't forget to remove the string after a day or so.)

Note: Remedies change as products change and improve. I recommend a visit to your local pharmacy (or friendly website) to check out the newest cures before you leave home. Test the ones you prefer, being certain you understand how to apply them. Better yet, check with a medical expert. Sports medicine specialists and podiatrists can be especially helpful.

TIP : 9.2 PREVENTION IS STILL THE BEST TREATMENT

- Wear high-quality, well-fitted boots (broken in, but not broken down) with insoles, wicking sock liners, and trekking socks. (See Step Two, "Gearing Up.")

- When you have a choice of surfaces, walk on softer ones. For example, choose the verge instead of pavement, leaves instead of stones.

- Keep your feet dry. Lightly powder or apply antiperspirant to the soles of your feet before putting on your liners.

- Reduce friction on blister-prone areas. Apply a lubricant or petroleum jelly to reduce chafing.

- When you stop to rest, weather and time permitting, take off your boots and socks to air cool and dry your feet.

Rainy Reflections

✤ J o u r n a l

Drenched

Before leaving on this walk, I promised myself that if Mike and I remained healthy and uninjured, I would be a good sport. I would not complain about rain, terrain, or minor inconveniences (like the damp sheets I slept between a few nights ago). Today, however, was so foul and so drenching, that complaining was justified. So, I'm giving myself a pass on my brief bout of whining. In a soaking rain, one spell of ill humor comes as close to "good sportsmanship" as this tenderfoot is likely to get. 🐾

DALES WAY DELUGE

It is day nine. Our last day. For an entire week we've been blessed with perfect fall weather. Only ten miles more to Bowness, a picturesque village on the shore of Lake Windermere.

Bowness, in the heart of England's Lake District, marks the end of the Dales Way, an eighty-six–mile trail across fields and fells, through centuries-old Yorkshire villages, along scenic rivers, and over more stone walls than my legs thought existed. Like hundreds of other off-road trails that cross the British countryside, the Dales Way is a rambler's dream come true. But today it is looking more like a nightmare. From the hallway window of the seventeenth century farmhouse where we've spent the night, I see dark clouds. I lace my boots and layer up for a rain pants/rain jacket/rain hood/pack cover day.

We bid farewell to Mrs. B, the farm wife who has been our host, as we step outside and take shelter under the cover of her porch. Mike, whose encouraging words have brought me this far, proclaims the cloud burst "just a passing cell." I feel reassured. After all, this is not the rain forest. This is England's Lake District. Surely, torrential rain can't last more than a few minutes. We wait.

Sheets of rain, pressed by gale-force winds, are soon blowing sideways across the porch. Confident, however, that the rain will soon abate, we set out. My clean, dry boots squish into the farm muck that covers Mrs. B's driveway. I walk by soggy cows waiting to be milked and border collies, tugging at their chains, eager to work in spite of the downpour.

Beyond the village of Burnside, we locate the trail we'll follow through the wet countryside. For the next five hours, I snap no photos to mark our drenching march to Bowness because my camera isn't waterproof. For lunch, I eat a damp energy bar. Only once do I respond to a biological imperative. Because only once do I feel desperate enough to do so. On this, our final day of tramping, England's pastoral quaintness remains a shadow behind a gauze of pelting rain.

Our progress is slow across slippery pastures dotted with sheep. Our glasses need wipers. Our boots need more waterproofing. Our layers stop breathing as sweat from inside merges with torrents from outside, and we tick off the miles of a head-down, get-through-it kind of day.

Still, we smile. Because we know how blessed we are to be healthy, to be able, to be together, to be holding a confirmed reservation at a bed and breakfast.

Our day ends at a cozy inn where towels and a hair dryer are waiting. The heat is on. The shower is hot. With our wet clothes draped over every horizontal surface, we sink into the luxury of clean, warm, and dry. Our journey has been accomplished, our bonds strengthened, our good sportsmanship confirmed.

KEEPING IT DRY

Rain offers a gradation of experiences for a walker, a continuum of wetness, from intermittent drizzle to torrential downpour. For every level of wetness, there is suitable (but seldom perfect) attire, from a rain jacket worn with or without a hood to rain pants worn over shorts or long johns.

For me, rainy day happiness depends on following three principles: first, every morning, everything I carry goes into plastic bags before it goes into my pack; second, my handy pack cover goes on my pack as soon as I feel the first rain drop—and sometimes sooner; and, third, I remind myself as I slog along that the hills and dales would not be dressed in the velvety green I love without the moisture that is falling on me.

TIP : 9.3 TRY FOR DRY

- Always wear your gaiters. Otherwise, water running down your legs will soak the insides of your boots.

- Put on your pack cover before your pack gets wet.

- Put on your rain gear before you get wet. It's easier to keep your clothes dry than to dry them later in a bedroom. (Not every B & B provides special drying facilities.)

- If you don't wear rain pants, the rain dripping off your jacket will wet your unprotected legs, shorts, or trousers.

- Carry a large plastic bag to use as a ground cover for your pack. It is also useful for sitting on after the rain stops (and for picnics on dry days, too).

- It's unfair, but on a warm, rainy day you won't be able to stay dry. You'll get wet either from rain or perspiration—or both.

- No matter how miserable you feel, you will eventually dry out.

- Be brave—rain doesn't last forever. Usually, not even a full day.

RAIN (AUTHOR UNKNOWN)

A poetic reminder that a walk can always get wetter…

It rained and it rained and rained and rained
The average fall was well maintained
And when the tracks were simply bogs
It started raining cats and dogs.

After a drought of half an hour
We had a most refreshing shower
And then the most curious thing of all
A gentle rain began to fall.

Next day was also fairly dry
Save for the deluge from the sky
Which wetted the party to the skin
And after that the rain set in.

Attitude Adjustment

Greetings

We're deep in canine country. Dogs meet and greet walkers all along the path. Today's collection included a springer spaniel trekking the entire Coast to Coast path with his humans, a brace of lurchers on their daily outing, and four sniffing, licking, dancing terriers.

A Jack Russell was part of the welcoming party at our B & B—a friendly, silly ratter who enjoys a soft berth. And, on our way to dinner, we met a border terrier off-lead that came running when called. Immediately. The first time he was called. Gambit is going to hear about this. ❧

PET THERAPY

After dragging myself over moorland atop the Pennines, my spirits need a lift. I look up from my boots and see it bounding my way on terrier paws—a wire-haired dog, panting with excitement, his carrot tail wagging wildly. He stops to balance on his hind legs and props his muddy front paws on my knees. Instant joy. Forgetting the twenty-three pounds secured to my back, I bend over (not a smart move) to return his effusive welcome and receive a lovely face lick. I'm relieved when I straighten up without difficulty.

"Name is Natty," comes a voice from the other end of the dancing dog's lead. "He's a good boy."

"I can see that! We miss our own little guy, who is a great greeter himself. A border terrier named 'Gambit.' He even has an English grandparent."

That's all it takes. We're off "talking dog," comparing notes, telling stories, making friends.

If you like animals, especially dogs (and cats and rabbits, too), the UK is a prime destination because you are never far from a furry face. In fact, the first sentence you're likely to hear at a B & B after "Please leave your boots outside" is, "This is Katie" (or Charlie, Suzie, Murphy, Woody, or some such). Katie, the official greeter swirling about your legs, is most likely a retired border collie, generic terrier, or friendly mixed-breed rescued from a shelter.

At a B & B in Cowgill on the Dales Way, Mrs. P invites us to hand feed other pets—her small herd of goats. Later, after a superb vegetarian evening meal, we retire to her living room. Mike plays an intense game of "catch-the-ring" with Jack, the resident border collie ("who has never liked sheep"), while I stroke the two resident lap-cats. There are no cows or sheep on the premises—originally built in 1660—because this B & B is not a farm. It's just a home with pet goats (and some ducks) in the backyard!

In pubs, too, we see dogs, but only if we look beneath the tables and bar stools where they like to curl up. Well-mannered and welcome, although a bit pungent in damp weather, they enjoy hanging out with their pub-mates. I have never heard a four-pawed patron bark.

A wagging tail is a pick-me-up on any path. Hug a furry new friend, and you forget tired feet, dense topo lines, and the miles ahead. Animal encounters fill homesick hearts, as they soothe and reassure, distract and strengthen. Such is the magic of licks and love.

TIP : 9.4 CANINE COMFORTS

- Dogs are numerous. Most are friendly.
- If one approaches on the trail, ask its human if you can pet it. If it seems especially friendly, you can probably pet it before asking.
- Move slowly and offer the back of your hand, knuckles first, for an investigative sniff.
- Ask about the dogs you meet on lead, in pubs, and in homes. Everyone likes "talking dog," especially when the subject is present.
- At your B & B, it's okay to address the dog first. The more fuss you make, the better.
- If you dislike, are allergic to, or are afraid of dogs or cats, you can avoid them, but with difficulty. Be sure to ask when you book your B & B whether a pet resides on the premises.

Grumpies

I've Had It

I'm struggling to put a lid on my whining. But I have a bad case of the "grumpies." My side hurts, and I'm tired and dragging. About a mile back, I was gazing at the downs–foot village of Fulking, instead of observing the ground beneath my feet, where I might have noticed that some adorable Rover had fouled the footpath. His mistake is now embedded in the tread of my right boot. Cow patties and sheep pellets may be unpleasant, but dog–do can undo one's day. And now, standing in the field we're about to cross is a hairy beast the size of a pick-up truck, with horns and a brass ring in his nose, looking mighty concerned about his turf. Mike is dressed in a red windbreaker. I start to grumble about things getting worse. 🐾

It's easy to focus on the inconsequential and the inconvenient, to feel frustrated about missing a waymark or inhabiting an upstairs bedroom so small and encrusted with knickknacks that not a speck of space is left to lay out a toothbrush.

For me, such foolish irritations pass quickly because, when the "grumpies" grab me, I turn my thoughts to Tom: Tom, who is my age and who once climbed mountains. Tom, who suffered a freak accident and now spends his days in a motorized wheelchair, paralyzed from his chest to his toes. Tom, whose determination inspires and whose spirit is undimmed. I think of Tom when the weather is too cold or too wet, the distance too long, and the hills too high to suit me. And when I do, I stop whining.

I put aside the "grumpies" and remember that it is a privilege to walk in the rain, even across a field guarded by a horned pick-up truck. I remember how fortunate I am to be able to place a foot into whatever fouls the footpath and to spend a claustrophobic night upstairs, in a bedroom cluttered with knickknacks. I remember and do not whine.

TIP : 9.5 Rx for Whiny Moments

- Write—Complaining into a journal can be as helpful as whining aloud, and it's easier on your travel mates. Writing about trials and tribulations invites perspective and is a safe way to ventilate feelings.

- Permission—Take five minutes while your feet are cooling or before lunch to BITCH. Do so forcefully, without inhibition, taking care not to blame your unhappiness on those traveling with you. Depending on the circumstances, you can rant publicly or in seclusion. Either way, you'll feel better, if not a little foolish. Just be sure to tell your listeners in advance that they're not responsible for fixing what's upsetting you, but that it would be nice if they would nod a few times and look sympathetic.

- Good sportsmanship—Maintaining a stiff upper lip is only required if you are British or in public. Otherwise, feel free to complain. But only briefly and not too often. Do it, enjoy it, get it over with, and move on.

- Sing—This works best when others join you in song.

- Smile—This simple action will lift your face and spirits at the same time. A smile is a reminder that there are always reasons to be happy—especially on a walk.

Mid-Soul

━━━━━━━━━━━━━━━━━━━━━━ ❦ Journal ━

Halfway

In the middle of a ramble, our approach to the pleasant miles we cover in long, easy strides and the hard ones we slog through becomes important. Because, like these miles, the ones we travel from youth to old age are middle ones. It is in the middle that we live our days. And it is here that we discover our happiness. ❦

The midpoint of a walk is technically the mile after which we have less distance ahead than we've already traveled. Sometimes it is just a feeling that a journey has started to wind down.

The midpoint is a sign that days and distances are decreasing. If we have not done so already, it reminds us to focus our attention on the countryside around us—this stile, that field, the next gray wall—and to worry less about reaching our destination.

Back home, I often ignore the beauty in life's middle moments. While selecting bright orange carrots in a grocery store, for example, I may be thinking about a prescription I need to fill at the pharmacy. While deadheading fragrant perennials in my garden, my thoughts may stray to what I should make for dinner. In the middle of a task, I'm too often somewhere else, my mind scanning my list of "things-to-do," while the color of carrots and the loveliness of flowers go unnoticed.

But when I walk, body and mind come together, especially after the midpoint of a path. After that divide, I think less about reaching the end (although a destination is a wonderful place to reach) and more about enjoying all the moments before I get there. As the days fall away and rambling becomes routine, the things that matter become clear: health, movement, comfort, safety, curiosity, discovery, beauty, direction, appreciation, awe, understanding, and friendship.

The middle of a walk is where we discover our rhythm and learn to relax and enjoy a path. We worry less about terrain, less about weather. We come to understand that the middle of a journey is where we feel most free and alive and where we usually have the most fun.

COMPETITIVE WALKING

A lean runner about our age slows down to walk with us. A determined sort of fellow, he tells us that he once ran the ninety-nine–mile path we're on in forty-eight hours. We are well aware that he probably ran more than ninety-nine miles because the distance a rambler covers normally exceeds "official" trail mileage by a considerable amount. Now, he's walking the same South Downs Way. This time at a "leisurely" pace—five days! (We plan to take nine.)

We also meet a power-walker wearing trainers (sneakers) and no socks. Dressed only in a tee shirt and shorts despite the brisk weather, he says he's training for this year's overnight race across the Downs. We can't keep up with either of these driven souls, although we try to do so for awhile because we'd like to continue our breathless conversations with them.

The soles of our own feet, protected inside sock liners, hiking socks, and sturdy boots, throb a bit after a day of walking on the sharp, chalky surfaces of the trail across the Downs. We wonder what it is that pushes these racers to punish their own bodies. Whatever it is, we don't have it.

Competitive walkers are a common sight in this green land where tramping is a national pastime. They're often trying to cover a specific distance in fewer hours, go more miles in a day, walk up more mountains, or accrue more lifetime miles than some mythical competitor. Who or what that competitor is, I'm not sure—perhaps some bloke in a pub back home, perhaps a previous record, perhaps their own aging bodies.

It's more likely, however, that they're simply drawn to one of the many competitive trials and tribulations that foster insanity in otherwise sane and sensible British walkers, and which have been devised to honor some tradition or past event. For example, they might enter the Yorkshire Three Peaks Challenge. This contest requires competitors to complete a grueling twenty-five-mile trek over the three highest peaks in Yorkshire, climbing a total of some 5,200 feet in less than ten hours.

Another temptation for the intrepid is the Lyke Wake Walk, a forty-mile trail across the North York Moors, on which coffins were once carried to the nearest (but often far-off) churchyard. Walkers who complete this distance in twenty-four hours qualify for a coveted membership in the fraternity of Lyke Wake Walkers.

Extreme walking invites injury and exhaustion. But it is irresistible to folks who engage in activities that many of the rest of us consider "over the top"—folks like our septuagenerian friend, Colin, who completed both of the above challenges and asserts, with a gleam in his eyes and a broad grin across his weathered face, that they were "great fun."

We, however, have no interest in competing. We don't "bag peaks" back home in the Adirondack Mountains. Nor do we race through our countryside walks, trying to cover the greatest distance in the fewest days. What drives us is the goal we've set for ourselves: *To experience a sense of place through intimate contact with the land and its people, while deriving the greatest pleasure per mile.*

On the South Downs Way, a path on which pilgrims, monks, drovers, and villagers once walked between Winchester and Canterbury, we stop, as we do on all our paths, to talk with other ramblers. All conversations eventually get around to the same question: "How many days will you be walking?"

At first we feel defensive about our obvious sloth and confess our tortoise-like plans with some discomfort. Surprisingly, our admission of "nine days" draws support and assurance.

"Very good, that. Nothing wrong with taking your time. Unfortunately, it's back to work for us on Monday."

Feeling better about our low "average daily mileage" and grateful that we don't have to hurry, we reply, "We're traveling at vacation speed. Going slowly so we can enjoy your beautiful countryside, your communities, and the path."

"Lovely. Best way to do it."

Who can argue with that?

Your Way Is Okay

I descend the stairs on a bright morning, sure-footed and athletic, carrying my pack, stick in hand. After six days of walking, I feel like an authentic rambler, ready to strut and stride over hill and dale.

"My, that's a very large rucksack for this path," says B & B host Barbara in a superior tone that momentarily deflates me.

"Not really," I counter. "I'm strong. Twenty-some pounds feels light to me. It only looks large because of the design of my pack. Here, look at the waist belt and…" I'm off chatting about my wonderful pack.

I will not let Mrs. Snooty-Put-Down steal my joy.

When I complete my "show and tell" defense of my belongings, Barbara claims to stand corrected, to have become more educated about packs and pounds. But I know she can't wait to tattle to her neighbors about those over-equipped Americans, who spent last night with her.

By then, however, I'll be miles away—well prepared for the weather, carrying what I need, striding over the next ridge.

- Don't let anyone intimidate you. "Know-it-alls" never do know it all.
- What suits you is what's best for you to wear and carry.
- Strength of conviction is as important as strength of muscle.
- Walk at your own speed in your own way.
- Know yourself. Choose your own path, and follow it.

Special Places

Journal

Stewards of the Land

I want to capture these vistas and take them home with me: broad, open areas dotted with farms; stone houses clustered into villages with markets and services that people reach by walking; and communities that value open space, serene beauty, and local history, all watched over by County Councils that seek to keep things the way they are.

I want the landscape back home to look like this. It's not that I don't see poverty and despair in the countryside. They're here in plain view. It's what I see in addition that connects me to this landscape: a vision of a future protected, a sense that much of what is here now will still be here when the children and grandchildren of today's ramblers put on their own rucksacks and strike out on a walk. 🌼

This is not the vision shared by people in the semi-rural region I call home. Open, undeveloped countryside there is vanishing and is almost entirely off-limits to the public. Where I live:

- Footpaths do not cross farm fields or golf courses, wend through private woodlands, or connect one community with another.
- There are virtually no rights-of-way or public footpaths across private property.
- Walking is mostly confined to trails in municipal and state parks and to town roads and city sidewalks.

- There is plenty of backcountry and wilderness hiking for rugged folks, who enjoy sleeping in tents and lean-tos, but not much walking for a tenderfoot who prefers indoor comforts near the trail at the end of an outdoor day.

- Farmers and other large landholders are transforming the landscape by selling acreage that has been protected by their families for generations. Their birthright is soon planted with mini-mansions and carved into cookie-cutter suburbs with streets named for natural things that once thrived on the land: Deer Run, Owl Lane, Woodland Drive, Forest Circle, Frog Hill, Orchard Terrace.

- Architectural guidelines have been abandoned to individual tastes, which, if local results are any indication, need some improving.

- Houses sprawl along roads and across what is left of open country, rather than clustering into villages, which are vanishing from the landscape.

- Towns, if they do survive, are seldom cozy or quaint—those that serve tourists excepted. Very few enjoy British amenities: pub, post office, school, library, church, green grocer, and public toilet. Not to mention: fish monger, butcher, cobbler, cheese monger, sweet shop, book shop, and bank. Instead, our smaller communities are reduced to self-service gas stations, convenience/video stores, and a main drag of franchises.

So it is not surprising that a tenderfoot, even one from a semi-rural, sparsely populated region, yearns to follow a real countryside path, a path that leads back across centuries. A path that travels where traditional architecture and human communities are valued and preserved, and where peace fills the heart and soothes the soul.

It is to such a footpath that this walker will return as often as possible for as long as possible.

Best Foot Forward
Trail-wise Trekking

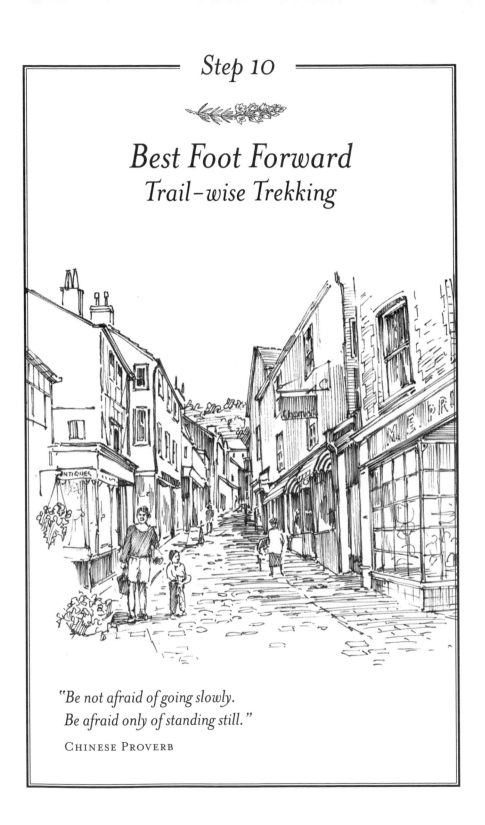

"Be not afraid of going slowly.
Be afraid only of standing still."

CHINESE PROVERB

Daily Doings

Pulse of the Path—Coast to Coast Walk

A Day Under Way—Offa's Dyke Path

Buddy System—The Cotswold Way

   TIP 10.1: It's Nice to Have a Buddy

Weather Wise—Coast to Coast Walk

Layered Breathing—South Downs Way

   TIP 10.2: Happy Layering

Pack Management—The Dales Way

   TIP 10.3: Packing Up

You Can Take It with You—Offa's Dyke Path

   JOURNAL: Temptation

   TIP 10.4: Memorabilia on Foot

   TIP 10.5: Going Postal

Squeaky Clean—Coast to Coast Walk

   TIP 10.6: Walker-Washed Laundry

When Nature Calls, We Must Answer

   JOURNAL: Relief

   When?

   Where?

   How?

   TIP 10.7: Pointers for Piddling

Naughty Nettle

The Nettle Way—Uphill to Old Harry

   TIP 10.8: Nettle Knowledge

Tips for the Tenderfoot

Tools

Keeping Comfy

Underway

Preventing Injury

Walking Maxims

In this chapter, as we walk across the countryside together, I'll be sharing my thoughts, personal experiences, and helpful tips. What may surprise you is that the aches, pains, and rain, which were our concern in Step Nine, are of little concern here as we march along, our heads held high, our serotonin levels buoyed by healthful exercise in natural landscapes and by human communities along the path.

I have selected personal stories and commentaries about "the basics" of rambling from seven wonderful, long-distance walks and mixed these with some practical advice. Armed with this information, you can set out with confidence, put your best foot forward, and anticipate success and satisfaction.

But first, we have these words from author Paul Millmore to give us his perspective on the rewards of a specific long-distance walk:

> In the late 20th century why would anyone want to walk or ride [a bike or horse] 99 miles…along the South Downs Way between Eastbourne and Winchester?
>
> There may be far easier methods of travel available but, to journey along this ancient route, away from the traffic, noise and dirt of the main roads, is an experience not to be missed… To step back in time, and voyage by simple means along this historic ridge top, is one of the best ways of reviving the spirit.
>
> …[T]here are so many sights to discover: Saxon and Norman churches, tumuli (the graves of settlers from over 3,000 years ago), medieval field systems where meager crops were grown, and dew ponds from the days of the huge 18th and 19th century sheep flocks.
>
> Seeing sheep still grazing the Downs and the butterflies feeding on the wild flowers gives the traveler a tremendous sense of continuity. High on the top of the dry, seamless hills you can get closer to the mind of the shepherd, pedlar or pilgrim who journeyed on this path centuries ago.
>
> The South Downs Way is a particularly attractive national trail for the uninitiated. You can quickly achieve a feeling of quiet isolation, even solitude, while actually staying close to civilisation.

Source: *South Downs Way*–National Trail Guide

Daily Doings

PULSE OF THE PATH — COAST TO COAST WALK

I love the day-after-day rhythm of walking. Each morning, we leave one B & B, and by evening, we arrive at another. Every day begins with a clear goal and ends with an accomplishment. Today's schedule resembles yesterday's, much like one sibling resembles another. Its pattern is familiar, but its unique attributes develop as time passes.

Each day acquires its own personality, depending on what is over head (rain, sun), in our faces (wind, splendid views), under foot (grass, mud, pavement), or on our backs (full packs or light ones). Today I'm feeling the extra weight of a packed lunch, fourteen postcards I still need to write, and a four-ounce badger knickknack I couldn't resist purchasing.

We set off from High Blakey, a small outpost with a pub and a B & B, located atop a high moorland ridge. A vicious wind howls across the treeless landscape, pushing us sideways. Planting our walking sticks to leeward, we press forward, trying to hold ourselves upright, using sinews strengthened over sixteen days of walking.

The wind intensifies and tosses me into the heather that, to my relief, is softer than the thorny gorse nearby. The spill injures my pride, but nothing else. Once I'm righted, we press steadily on, so anxious to get this nasty gale behind us, that we arrive early in Glaisdale, our safe harbor for the night.

There is nothing much to do in the village, but this doesn't matter. Arriving is what counts. And having done that, we're content. Another successful day. Another journey completed. Well done.

Tomorrow, the windstorm will have blown by. And we'll begin again.

A DAY UNDER WAY — OFFA'S DYKE PATH

9:30   Set out. Temperature in high fifties and rising. A day for shorts.

10:30   Rest stop. Take off pack. Remove long sleeve shirt. Change from ski hat to baseball cap. Drink water. Photo-op.

11:00	Perfect scenery. Rolling hills. Stop for a photo (one of a dozen or more photo stops throughout the day).
1:00	Rest time. Pack off. Drink more water. Eat a light lunch: Scottish shortbread, energy bar, toast and jam saved from breakfast, and a piece of fruit. High-carb heaven.
1:20	Hit the trail. Temperature in mid-seventies.
2:00	Stop to talk with walkers going in the opposite direction, led by a border terrier that looks like our dog, Gambit. Receive a canine greeting. Drink more water.
2:15	Back to business. Time to walk.
3:15	Rest stop. Put on long sleeve shirt. Take another picture. Drink more water.
4:00	Arrive at B & B. Enjoy a "nice cuppa," along with some Welsh tea cakes.
5:00	Retreat to room. Rest, bathe, do hand wash, "dress" for dinner.
6:30	Leave for pub.
9:30	Return to B & B. Too tired to write postcards. Write a few words in journal. Read a few words in guidebook. Fall fast asleep.

Buddy System — The Cotswold Way

The day is cool as we leave Painswick in a light rain. An hour later, after a prolonged climb, I reach my saturation point—wetter inside from perspiration than outside from rain. I'm getting a mite cranky when the sun rescues me, and I decide to shed my sodden layers.

This is a great time to have a buddy. Mike holds my pack above the puddles while I wriggle out of it and unfold a plastic bag to create a dry spot to set down both our packs. I store my rain gear and then "un-layer" down to a tee shirt and shorts. Mike lifts my pack again to return it to my shoulders, after which I help him with his.

At these and other moments, especially on hard days, and because I like to talk, I'm aware that I could not travel happily without a buddy. If Mike were not interested in walking, and if I couldn't persuade a girlfriend to walk with me, an organized tour would be my alternative. In a group, someone is always there to offer assistance and share conversation.

The buddy system is a useful arrangement because two arms may not be enough to lift and carry things, and because two heads are more fun than one when sharing impressions, complaints, and pints of bitter. And because there is nothing like having a buddy at your side when you're feeling a little lost.

TIP : 10.1 It's Nice to Have a Buddy
- To reach into your pack and hand you what you need.
- To help you remove your pack without straining your back.
- To share your challenges and triumphs.
- To take your picture.
- To stop, look, and listen when you say, "Oh, just look at that."
- To ease your aches and pains with reassurance.
- To help figure out directions when you think you're lost.
- To join you in song.
- To help wring out wet laundry in dry towels.
- To watch your pack when you visit a store or public toilet.
- To remember the journey with you after you return.

Being your own buddy can also be pleasant. Walking in solitude, away from chatter (even if only for an hour), clears the mind and frees the spirit. At the end of a solitary ramble, a walker, feeling refreshed and restored, will be ready once again to socialize and reconnect with friends and family.

Weather Wise — Coast to Coast Walk

Engulfed in fog, I long for the familiar voice of NOAA (U.S. Government) weather radio. I'd even embrace the overly exuberant meteorologist/entertainer on the early news back home if he could shed some light on our situation and tell us when this fog will lift and our footpath reappear.

I'm homesick for a detailed weather report, hungry for the in-depth analysis I take for granted in U.S. forecasts. In a land where news is covered in detail on telly and radio morning and evening, weather reporting is often treated as an afterthought. Although better and more detailed than in the past, forecasts are mostly brief, general, and delivered at twice the speed of normal speech. Why is this? Perhaps the British public doesn't care if it gets slapdash forecasting of conditions pertinent to walkers. Apparently, vague information is good enough. "You don't understand," they assert. "This is an island nation. The weather is always changing."

"True enough," I reply. "But doesn't anyone care in which direction it's changing? Doesn't British Airways or the military care? Don't they need accurate forecasts? Wouldn't they like to share some details with the rest of us?"

As we make our way from Kirkby Stephen to Keld, we don't know if, or when, the fog will lift. We don't know if dampness will give way to rain or sunshine. Scrambling across wet upland bogs, we have no idea whether this bitter day will warm up or remain in the grip of a cold front. On the radio this morning, the rapid-fire, unhelpful forecast was for "a bit of a damp start to the day." One glance out the window, and I knew as much myself. Stuck in the foggy present, we haven't a clue about the future. And given the current state of forecasting, it looks like foggy facts are all we're likely to get.

LAYERED BREATHING — SOUTH DOWNS WAY

Today has been another hard-to-dress-for day. I start out wearing my usual nylon "relaxed" tights and a polyester tee shirt. Over my tee, I layer a long sleeve shirt and a lightweight fleece zip-up turtleneck. I put on gloves and a bright pink ski hat. An hour later, I take off my pack and replace my fleece outer layer with a featherweight wind shell. While my pack is resting, I visit the bushes to answer nature's call. Ready at last, I put on my pack. My layers are breathing nicely.

By 10:30 my hat is marginal. Downhill and into the wind, it's toasty perfection. But uphill and downwind, it's too warm. I hand the hat to Mike, who stuffs it into the top of my pack along with my gloves. He hands me the pink baseball cap that is attached to my pack with a carabiner. The sun is growing stronger.

At 11:30 it's time for another pack-off moment—staying hydrated has its downside. It's also time to remove more layers. I put away my long sleeve shirt and my wind shell and continue walking in long pants and a tee shirt. I think about changing into shorts, but decide I can wait. With Mike's assistance, I put on my pack again.

This arrangement works until lunch. Sitting on a ridge top, overlooking a downs-foot village and the trail stretching miles ahead, I am chilly the moment the wind touches my damp body. I reach for my fleece hat and zip-up turtleneck for the second time today. Instant warmth.

All is comfy until we are ready to carry on. Off come the protective layers. I shiver. On goes my pack. My back feels warmer. Fortified with calories and enthusiasm, we move as swiftly as we are able after a proper lunch. Within minutes short sleeves, which were too cold for sitting, are just right for walking.

As the sun descends and the wind rises, we stop again to add layers. And so it goes. Not every day is like this, but many are. At the end of these pack on/pack off, zip up/zip down days, I like to reward myself with a second serving—let us say, an extra layer—of apple crumble or chocolate cake for dessert.

Tip : 10.2 Happy Layering

- Don't suffer. Layer up or down before you get chilled or overheated.

- Don't worry about time. It takes fewer than five minutes to remove your pack, take off a layer, stow it, and replace your pack.

- Don't hesitate. As soon as it starts to rain, put on your rain gear and pack cover. Once you're wet, it's too late to stay dry.

- Start out cooler than is comfortable. Walking will warm you.

- Add a layer when you stop walking. Sitting still will cool you.

- Standing around when it's breezy and cloudy will also cool you.

- Uphill is warmer than downhill. Downhill is warmer than stationary. Calm is warmer than windy.

- The warmth of a sunny day lightens loads and lifts spirits. Cherish every day you can walk in a tee shirt and shorts, even if you have to carry the weight of your extra layers.

Pack Management — The Dales Way

The promise of another beautiful day in the Dales shines through our bedroom window as bells toll in the tower of the old Norman church beyond the gate. We are busy rolling our clothing and accessories into plastic bags, shoving the softest and lightest of them into the bottoms of our packs. The scent of coffee and grilled mushrooms seeps into our nest, urging us to hurry. It will not do to be late for the first, and often best, meal of an English day.

Our B & B, a tiny private house, was vacated for us by its owners who spent the night with a daughter, who lives nearby. The activity in the kitchen tells us that our hosts have returned to prepare breakfast while we collect our gear. We force ourselves to work slowly, taking care to pluck what is ours from among the wall-to-wall knickknacks and antiques (two from the days of Roman occupation) that occupy every shelf, table, and corner.

I'm becoming quite efficient at the daily ritual of emptying the contents of my pack at night into organized piles on a bedroom floor, and then reversing the routine in the morning to repack my stacks of possessions.

At the moment I have a dilemma. I've kept out my toothbrush, toothpaste, and dental floss to use after breakfast. But I'd like to place these into my toiletries kit and bury that about halfway down in my pack, cover it with the rest of my things, and tighten my compression straps in preparation for a quick, post-breakfast getaway. Shall I brush now and finish my packing? Or brush later and close up after breakfast? If I had a luggage transfer service, this would be a moot point. But I don't. And it isn't.

I decide to brush now, pack my dental supplies, and shove my kit into the center of my pack to prepare for a hasty exit after breakfast. (I will rinse my mouth to assuage my dental guilt.) The sun is shining, and I don't want to waste a minute of this glorious day.

Tip : 10.3 Packing Up

- Empty your pack each evening.
- In the morning, smooth out the duvet that kept you cozy all night. On it lay out ALL your belongings.

- Check under beds and between knickknacks for stray socks and laundry.
- Pack up as soon as you can—before breakfast if possible. If your B & B is cold and you need to wear extra layers to endure a cold dining room, then pack right after breakfast.
- Always check the room again before departing. Did you remember your water bottle, the hat you hung on the back of the door, your toothbrush in the bathroom, your sandwich, walking stick, and travel alarm clock?

You Can Take It with You—Offa's Dyke Path

=== ❧ J o u r n a l ===

Temptation

Why can't I resist a souvenir like the cardboard beer mat (coaster) under my half-pint of ale? It will look great in our album. All I have to do is get it home without bending it. Still, I'm hesitating, even though "it weighs hardly anything," because I've said that about each of the postcards I collected, the decorative map I had to have, and the tiny insect pins tucked deep into my pack. And since English notes in denominations less than five-pounds-sterling don't exist, I have also accumulated a number of heavy coins. Taken together, these things are beginning to weigh me down. I've also added six pieces of dark chocolate. Happily, in six days these will be gone. And then I won't even notice the cardboard coaster. ❧

Arriving in Knighton shortly after noon to enjoy a half-day of leisure, we find our hostess to be both accommodating and gracious. Mrs. S brews some tea for Mike and me and a French press of coffee for Robin. She sets these and a plate of biscuits on a table for us to enjoy in the warmth of her walled garden. An hour later, revived, refreshed, and pack free, we set off to explore the town and its shops. Such is the joy of a free afternoon.

Our first stop is Canolfan Clawdd Offa (Offa's Dyke Centre), the "official" halfway point on the trail and the headquarters and retail outlet for the Offa's Dyke Association. Its historical exhibits are captivating, but its souvenir pickings are slim. I don't need a sweatshirt, tee shirt, or another book to carry. At the rate I've been reading (one page a night before unconsciousness), the slim, used book I purchased for one pound in Hay-on-Wye will last our entire journey.

What I really want is something small and light—something like a lapel pin or a replica of the coin struck by King Offa over 1,100 years ago. The coin had his likeness on it, and I'd like one to carry for good luck.

Reluctantly, I settle for an assortment of memorabilia that, when taken together, does not meet my needs the way a single, but unavailable, coin would have done. I purchase bookmarks, pens, and a tiny metal shield to attach to my wooden walking stick back home. I also buy four postcards for our album and six more I intend to write this evening—if I stay awake long enough.

My collection of nonessentials in hand, we proceed to the post office, purchase a mailing envelope, and send our assorted trinkets home on a slow boat.

We are ready now to inspect the shops. But we can't. Not in Knighton. Not on Wednesday. In Knighton, Wednesday is "half-day closing," the bane of visitors to rural Britain. Following a tradition most likely held over from the Middle Ages, many towns still select one weekday (usually Wednesdays) to close their shops at noon (food stores, bakeries, pubs, and pharmacies generally excepted). It is very unlikely, but you could walk an entire path, and find stores shut for "half-day closings" whenever you have a free afternoon.

Across from the post office, a closed sporting goods store displaying quality gear and souvenirs catches our attention. In its window there is a small sand-casting I could die for: a "must-have" figurine of a border terrier, impossible to find back home. Next to it are three small pewter pins that call to me—a dragonfly, a lizard, and a turtle. A sign on the door says the store will reopen Thursday at 9 AM, after we plan to be on our way.

I explain to my fellow walkers that the goods before me are essential to my well-being (this from someone who hates to shop) and that I will regret forever leaving without them. Then I say, "We really need to stop back here in the morning. Is a late start doable?"

"Of course. No problem." A late start, they know, is better than miles of whiny regrets.

At 8:58 Thursday morning we are standing in front of the store when the proprietor arrives, looking rested from her half-day off. Minutes later, the treasures are mine, wrapped and ready for the post office across the street. I stash the pewter pins into my pack where they join yesterday's postcards and the dark chocolates I bought in Kington two days ago. I intend to wear the dragonfly tonight when I "dress" for dinner. Carrying this extra weight will be a pleasure.

All day Mike talks about another figurine we left behind in the window, a sweet lamb resting on a pair of hiking boots, a tableau of British walking. I know "consumer regret" when I hear it. So, at 4 PM, when we arrive at our hilltop B & B, I call the shop in Knighton. It's open. No early closing today.

"Yes, of course I remember you, the shopkeeper replies after I introduce myself. "Yes, it's still here. In the window. Very good. Shall I wrap it and send it to you in the States? Right. I'll take care of it. Have a good walk."

Aren't credit cards and telephones wonderful?

We are both content. We have what we want. And when we get home, a resting lamb and a little border terrier will share our kitchen and our memories for many years. Brilliant.

Tip : 10.4 Memorabilia on Foot

- If you're using a luggage transfer service, or if you're on a tour, the sky is almost the limit for acquiring souvenirs. You only have to carry your purchase until you meet up with your luggage in the evening or with a tour leader, who can take the treasure off your hands or out of your pack.

- If you are on your own, feel free to purchase a gift, as long as you can carry it to the nearest post office. There you can buy wrapping/packaging supplies and mail it home to yourself.

- Carry with you in your pack the tiny gifts you love, as long as they add more to your walk than just their weight.

- As your walk progresses, you'll grow stronger. So don't worry about adding a few light mementos to your pack. When you get home, the weight will have been worth it.

- What you decide to carry with you depends on the space in your pack and the pounds on your back. Our friends Bob and JoAnne, who did the Coast to Coast Walk, trekked the last fifty miles of it carrying a bottle of Champagne, which they expected to open, but didn't until they got home. Then they opened it to celebrate (with us) the completion of their walk.

- When you return to base camp and your overseas luggage, you can shop with abandon. And if you're still carrying them, you can also write those postcards you intended to send along the way. Just remember to post them before leaving for home.

TIP : 10.5 GOING POSTAL

- Classic British red post boxes are still in use but can be difficult to find. One we nearly missed was hidden within a stone wall and covered in ivy. They make great backdrops for photos and are convenient drop-offs for postcards.

- If you want your postcards to reach the States in days rather than weeks, affix airmail stamps and stickers to them. (In Britain, there is a big difference between regular and air-mail.) You can purchase stamps in many stores and hotels, as well as in all post offices.

- Buy a few extra stamps and stickers for mailing postcards en route.

- Take along preprinted address labels or a light address book. Seal these inside a small plastic bag, along with your stamps and stickers.

- Many post offices are located in stores where you can also purchase supplies for wrapping and taping packages to send home.

SQUEAKY CLEAN—COAST TO COAST WALK

Our hotel in Orton is a laundry bonanza. As we check in, I ask Patrick, the man in charge of everything, for extra towels and a few tablespoons of laundry powder. As is our daily custom, we are planning to wash out a few things in our room sink before dinner.

I need the soap powder because our room is supplied with liquid body wash—no bar soap. (No shampoo either.) I need towels because after I wring out my underwear, sock liners, and tee shirt, Mike and I, working together, will roll these items into a spare towel and wring them out again to remove as much moisture as we can before draping them over a length of parachute chord, which we carry for this purpose, or over towel racks—many of which are heated in Britain.

Laundry is a top priority on our agenda. We do it as early as we can, almost always before dinner, to give our clothes plenty of time to dry. Patrick, however, has a better idea. For a few pounds, he will be happy to do our wash for us—all our wash. In this respect, we've been lucky. About every five days or so, we seem to arrive at a laundry oasis: a B & B or inn with a willing proprietor, a working washing machine, and a functioning dryer or handy clothesline.

We accept Patrick's unbeatable offer, remove ourselves to our room, and peel away our ripening inner and outerwear. We collect shirts, trousers, and thick hiking socks, along with the personal apparel we've been washing out nightly in sinks of assorted sizes with slow drains.

The pile of fermenting garments on the floor would constitute about half a load of laundry at home. Here, it will be two loads. At home, our wash is in a hot dryer fewer than thirty minutes. In England, it might toss about for an hour or more, unless there is a warm room indoors or the weather is fine. Then damp clothing is granted a reprieve and is pegged on a line.

Before handing over the only clothes we have in the world for our walk, I separate our pile into dark-colors and everything else. I ask Patrick to use cool or warm water, a low dryer setting, and please, "NO fabric softener." I ask him to call me when the wash is done and before he places anything in the dryer because I would like to air dry our more delicate items in our room.

I know better than to raise my expectations. I assume our clothes are destined to receive a "proper" wash and that I'm destined to be ignored. Blacks and whites will tumble together in hot water with added fabric softener before they are transferred to a dryer without anyone alerting me to retrieve the underwear and wool socks I prefer to air dry.

Surprisingly, our clothes—so far—have been able to endure this kind of repeated abuse and have survived to walk another day (a credit to their makers), perhaps a bit worse for wear and washing, but still functional. Rather like us. Up to the challenge and likely to reach the end of this journey in one piece.

At 9 PM Patrick rings. He has completed our wash. I tramp down to the front desk and pay a few pounds for the fragrant, warm bundle as Patrick explains, "Sorry this is late. I cranked up the dryer to its hottest setting, and it still took three cycles to finish your clothing."

"Right," I say, worried now about what remains of our quick-drying garments. "Thanks for finishing them."

TIP : 10.6 WALKER-WASHED LAUNDRY

The best feature about this do-it-yourself option is its predictable, timely result. So dip in, get your hands wet, and have some fun.

· Do your wash as early as you can after arriving at your B & B. Air drying in damp weather may take longer than you expect. When possible, hang your wash in a warm drying room or on an outdoor line in the sunshine.

· Each evening, wash the layers closest to your skin (especially your sock liners) to keep them wicking properly. Washing prevents dirt from filling the fabric's pores and grinding your liners to shreds.

· Wash your hiking socks every few days. Do this early enough to give them a chance to dry. Happily, today's modern wool blends can usually survive a dryer when one is available.

· Pack a flat, rubber sink stopper. British sink stoppers are unreliable.

· Ask your host for some washing powder (if there is only body wash or shower gel in your room) and for a few extra towels (not from her matching guest set). Wring out your laundry by hand. Then use a towel to wring it out again.

· When a dryer or a clothesline is not handy, your belongings will have to dry in your room overnight. This is why it is best to walk in quick-drying clothing that can stand up to washing machines and dryers.

· Remember that standards of cleanliness on a walk are relative and are useful only when they are flexible.

Relief—Offa's Dyke Path

I emerge from the shrubbery. Mike is holding my pack to reduce my effort and time getting back into it. He still hopes that someday I'll be able to execute a FAST pit stop—one like his. But nothing is fast when a female stops to piddle. It takes five to seven minutes, no matter how much she hurries. By now, he and Robin, our British walking companion, are used to waiting patiently. While I'm about my business, they have time to rest, review the trail guide, and check GPS data.

At least I think they wait patiently while I'm busy in the heather. They never complain. And why should they, blessed as they are with anatomy designed for outdoor adventure? With their equipment, they can piddle almost anywhere. They can do so quickly and discretely with their packs on, standing comfortably, gazing into the distance.

"Okay," I say after drinking another eight ounces of water, ensuring that we'll be stopping again before too long. "Thanks for waiting. Let's hit the trail." To which I add, because I can't resist, "Wagons ho." I think I see them smile. 🦋

On a walk I do not worry about natural bodily functions. Stimulated by a hearty English breakfast and daily exercise, assisted by lots of fluids, and perhaps a glass of ale at day's end, I have found that morning (or evening) visits to the loo for "number two" become predictable and routine. The real issue underway, particularly for females, is piddling. So let me address three frequently asked questions about this occasionally urgent subject.

When?

I pause to piddle whenever the need arises, as soon as I can find a convenient spot. My first stop is usually an hour or two after starting out each morning (often when I remove my first layer of clothing), followed by two or three more stops throughout the day. Frequency depends on my "drink-it-in, sweat-it-out" ratio. When this is in balance, there are not many reasons to stop. But, even if I don't feel the need, whenever I take my pack off to rest, snack, or alter layers, I also take time to piddle.

Piddling underway, however, is not a universal practice. One woman I know, who is an avid walker, rarely relieves herself underway. She says that she would if she needed to, but that nature never calls. I suspect that if her fluid intake were higher or her pack had a hip belt that cinched across her bladder as mine does, nature might call her more often.

She has accompanied me off trail, providing privacy for me by shielding me from view, without the slightest inclination to relieve herself and take pity on her own bladder. I have seen water go into her, but have rarely known it to come out during a day of walking. It appears that nature calls her only when a real, honest-to-goodness loo is present. Needless to say, her male partner doesn't suffer from such inhibition.

Where?

Almost anywhere with a modicum of privacy will do, as long as it is not uphill from a brook or pond you might pollute. Even a wide open space is fine if no other walkers are in sight. Unlike urban settings, where restrooms in stores and offices are reserved, locked, and unavailable, the great outdoors is an "equal relief" opportunity open to all.

I have piddled in grouse butts and bracken. I have piddled while braced against fence posts, Roman ruins, and cast-off, rusted, farm machinery. I'd rather not piddle hidden among prickly gorse (although I did this once), nor anywhere close to stinging nettle (I've done this more than once). Nor do I piddle along narrow roads bordered by hedges. Cars invariably appear on cue.

In many towns, there are public restrooms. Most are clean. Ditto for toilets at campsites and parks. And should we pass an open pub, I always ask to use the loo. I have never been refused.

How? (Males may skip this section.)

I carry something I call a "piddle pack" in my pocket. (Woe be to the walker without pockets.) It is a plastic zip-sealed sandwich bag. In it I place moist towelette packets, tissues or toilet paper, and another small plastic bag. I no longer carry sanitary products, although I once did in the days before hot flashes, when I had fewer wrinkles, more energy, and thicker bones.

I select a suitably private spot and remove my backpack, leaving it on the trail in Mike's care. Unless you are carrying a light day pack, it is easier on your back if you remove your pack before answering nature's call. Unencumbered, you can easily venture off the path to address your needs.

I take care to face downhill in order to keep my boots and vulnerable clothing dry and because it is easier to balance turned in this direction. When finished, I use a tissue, wash up with a towelette if necessary, place the used items in the empty bag, and return everything to my plastic, zip-sealed piddle pack. Done.

In the evening, I empty the paper wastes from the inner bag into a trash can—never into a "plumbingly challenged," British loo. Then I either wash out or replace the used (inner) trash bag, replenish my paper supplies, and I'm ready for the next day. Ready to hydrate without hesitation, to answer nature's call, and to ramble on in comfort.

TIP : 10.7 POINTERS FOR PIDDLING

Piddle when you must.
Piddle when you can.
Piddle whenever you stop for other reasons.
Piddle even in the rain. It may be unpleasant, but not piddling is worse.

· Think FUN. Your bladder works better, and you play better when you're both relaxed.

· For females:
  – Remove your pack before proceeding, especially if it's heavy.
  – Carry a "piddle pack." (See description above.)
  – If at first you don't succeed, try again. Do not get discouraged. With a little practice, a shy bladder will learn to do what comes naturally and piddle "al fresco."

· For males:
  – Piddling is easier in trousers designed with flies, especially if your pack has a hip belt.
  – Wind direction and velocity really matter.

Naughty Nettle

Stinging nettle, which grows along many footpaths in Europe, is a harmless but irritating plant with rather large leaves. The plant is called "stinging" because if you brush by it or sit in it (sooner or later you'll do both), your skin will redden and feel like it's under attack from dozens of needles and pins. The tingle, or burning sensation usually doesn't last long (from a few minutes to an hour or so), but it will get your attention. Happily, relief is often close by.

Look around, and you are likely to find a plant called dock, a walker's friend, growing close to the nettle that "stung" you. (Refer to a wildflower guide, or go on-line, to identify both dock and stinging nettle.) If you tear off a leaf from the dock, crush it a bit, and rub it briskly on your tingles, it will help soothe your skin. In a few minutes, you'll feel well enough to stop swearing.

The Nettle Way — Uphill to Old Harry

Muddy bridleway tracks and missing waymarks would have made today's fourteen-mile walk from Wells to Castle Cary a challenge even without the stinging nettles that covered the stiles and obscured the footpath.

We set out from our B & B in Wells at 9:30 to visit the city's renowned cathedral. By 11:00 we are heading south on the fifth day of an autumn ramble across Somerset and Dorset. Our route combines several regional paths, each with its own name. But after today, our footpath will forever be known to us as the "Nettle Way."

All day a plague of nettles nips at our heels, arms, and legs, while the dock that we need to soothe its stings remains scarce. I grab a leaf of dock when I do find one and tuck it away to apply later, after the next nettle attack. Tomorrow I may wear trousers.

In over a decade of walking, we have never seen such an abundance of stinging nettle and other dense vegetation, much of it armed with thorns. Robin, our British walking companion, theorizes that an unusually wet summer is to blame for the green explosion. But I'm convinced that neglected path maintenance is to blame. I posit very loudly—and quite often—that our so-called "trail" has yet to confront the blades of pruning shears (secateurs) or a weed trimmer this year.

The overgrowth, however, does give way to Robin's two walking sticks, which he brandishes like the swords of a knight in battle. Pausing at each jungle-covered stile, Robin beats back the worst of the nettles and clears the stile's posts and steps. Over we go, trying to avoid "the ones that got away," before moving forward, knee-deep in unpruned plant material.

As we bushwhack along a muddy woodland track, we are looking forward to the open pastureland and groomed trails, which we hope we'll find just ahead. The sun warms us as we climb gentle hills and try to ignore the gauntlet of stings and scratches. Happily, with Robin's walking sticks at the ready and our B & B getting closer, we manage to do what any walker would do. We search for dock, rub our wounds, and carry on.

TIP : 10.8 NETTLE KNOWLEDGE

- Try as you might to avoid it, stinging nettle will probably reach out and touch you.
- Its discomfort is tolerable and usually doesn't last long.
- If you rub a nettle sting with a leaf of dock, your tingles will diminish and may even disappear.
- Dock commonly grows close to nettles.
- An encounter with stinging nettle distinguishes you as a "true countryside walker." So wear your tingles proudly.

Tips for the Tenderfoot

What follows is an assortment of personal suggestions from this and other chapters to help make your *stepping out* vacation easy and pleasant. Why learn the hard way—from experience—when a list will do? The one below is an eclectic collection of favorite ideas from a tenderfoot, who has been where you are going.

TOOLS

- Maps are essential. Use an Ordnance Survey map, trail guide, strip map, or a combination. Use a GPS device if you are so inclined. Don't rely on waymarks. They may not be present when you need them. And they almost never give mileage.

- Keep your camera handy.
- Place items you might need during your day of walking near the top of your pack, in an exterior pocket, or in a handy pouch attached to your pack straps.

KEEPING COMFY
- If you can, walk on soft surfaces and avoid rocks.
- Take time out to remove your socks and cool your hot feet, especially while your soles are adapting to new demands.
- Place a folded fleece sock, or something equally soft, under each of your shoulder straps, even if the straps are padded.
- Piddle whenever you have an opportunity, even if you don't think you need to do so—meaning whenever your pack is off and you have a bit of shelter, or you pass a public restroom. You don't know when you'll have another chance.
- Schedule a rest day, or a half-day of walking, into your plans for a change of pace and to give yourself time to relax and explore.
- Often it is not the miles you walk per day that make you tired, but the weight of your pack and the number of hours you carry it.
- Plan to arrive at your B & B early on most days. Between 3 and 4 PM is good. If you can, let your hosts know when to expect you.
- If an evening meal is available, arrange in advance to have dinner at your B & B. This arrangement is convenient, and you won't be disappointed.

UNDERWAY
- Take your time going over stiles. They can be slippery. Use your poles to help you balance. Remember, a turtle carrying a pack is not as graceful as a hare dressed in a svelte jogging suit.
- When going over a stile, watch for barbed wire. Do not touch it. Do not allow your pack to touch it. Proceed with caution. If you don't clear it, it could rip your clothing, your pack, or you.
- Footing is important. Notice where and how you place your feet.
- You can eat wild blackberries. But resist the temptation along busy

roads, farm boundaries, and in other areas sprayed with chemicals or likely to be "marked" by dogs.

- Expect to meet dogs. Expect them to greet you.

PREVENTING INJURY

- Rambling does not lend itself to multitasking. When you come to a glorious scene, *stop* before you *look*.
- Remember, you are wearing a pack and you weigh more than usual. Be good to your knees and back. Avoid twisting. Bend and kneel with care.
- Stretch a little before putting on your pack each morning and after removing it each evening.
- Move like a gazelle—with graceful strides and fluid motion—as often as the terrain and your mood allow.

WALKING MAXIMS

- When you come to a critical fork on an otherwise well-marked path, the waymark will be missing. (Time to check your map.)
- The trail that goes uphill is probably yours.
- You won't realize that you've lost the path until you've walked uphill a mile or so from where you went astray.
- A ramble downhill will be followed by a trudge uphill. Eventually, you regain elevation you lose—probably when you're tired.
- You'll be hot going uphill and chilly on top.
- You cannot avoid cow patties and sheep droppings on grazed land.
- Muck and mud are unavoidable—even in dry weather—especially on bridleways and around farm gates.
- The pub you see just off your path will be closed for lunch.
- Every B & B is a welcome sight at the end of an active day.
- The first morning you do not thoroughly check your room, you will leave your toothbrush behind.
- It's easy to feel happy on a walk.

Okay. You're ready. Walk with joy. And let your spirit soar.

Walk in Progress
Comments from the Path

*"It takes time and trouble to persuade
ourselves that the things we want to do
are the things we ought to do."*

AGNES REPPLIER (1855–1950)

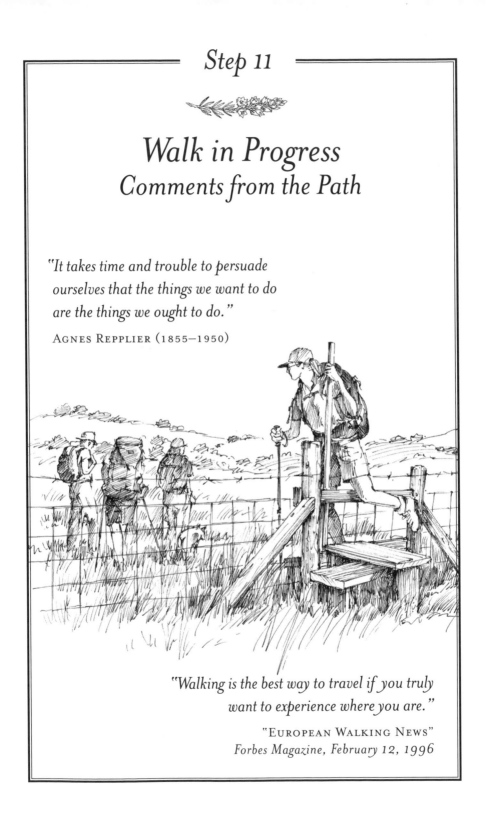

*"Walking is the best way to travel if you truly
want to experience where you are."*

"EUROPEAN WALKING NEWS"
Forbes Magazine, February 12, 1996

Day In, Day Out

Single-Tasking
Offa's Dyke Path: Llandegla to Llangynhafal

I swear I will never multitask again in an attempt to compress the lists of things I should do, but don't have time to do, and may never do. "To-do" lists create guilt, and multitasking leaves me depleted.

This morning, after I put on my pack and head down the path or up the first hill, I will be focused on only one thing, the only item on today's to-do list: walk. That's it. Simple. Doable.

On a ramble, multitasking is reduced to walking while snacking or while listening to the stories of others, with time-outs for stopping to check a map, take a drink, or snap a photo of a Welsh farm in the valley below.

I am learning as I walk to concentrate my attention on the here and now—an act that evokes simple pleasures. When was the last time I felt so focused and so satisfied? ※

Perfect Day
Coast to Coast Walk: St. Bees to Cleator

Walking at last. Our first real day of vacation. Already I feel at home in England. I am awake, alive, comfortable—engaged in the simplicity of walking. So far, only my smile muscles hurt. If only all days were like this one.

Today I am Goldilocks. Things are "just right." Last night's B & B was flawless. I don't have a single suggestion to offer when we depart after a night of sound sleep. We step out into sunlight, wearing fresh clothing, not an ache or pain to trouble us, on this, the first day of our Coast to Coast walk.

We take a photo of the sign that marks the start of our cross-country path and head to the beach a few yards beyond to honor a tradition. We dip the toes of our boots into the Irish Sea, our hopes high that nineteen days and two hundred miles from now, we will dip them into the North Sea at the end of our journey.

The weather is windy, but remains warm and dry. When nature calls, I am able to locate convenient, private places to answer. My pack is not as light as I would like, but at twenty-three pounds it seems sensible. As far as I can tell, nothing I'm wearing is chafing. Waymarks appear when we need them to confirm questionable information on our strip map. We move forward with confidence along a lovely path with views of the sea.

At Cleator, Pat, our B & B hostess, joins us for tea and suggests that we take our evening meal at a restaurant a short walk from her home. Our dinner, as promised, is outstanding—five kinds of steamed vegetables, perfectly roasted lamb, and an ultra-dark chocolate custard. We linger two hours to celebrate the end of this perfect first day before returning to our comfortable, spacious room and Pat's relatively modern plumbing.

Tomorrow, I fear, will be different. With the forecast calling for foul weather, we expect to make a withdrawal from the contentment we deposited today. We have fourteen miles to walk, which will probably be in showers and high winds. At night our escape from the elements will be a remote youth hostel with no power or heat. Dread is spreading through me like an oil slick.

But I am determined to remain in this lovely moment, in the present, where my bed is warm, the day still perfect, and I can think about how lucky I am to have lived it. ⚜

TIP : 11.1 NOT QUITE PERFECT

- Perfection, like truth and beauty, is seldom evident in our imperfect lives. Glitches are a given.
- Even on the best of days, things seldom go as smoothly as we wish.
- When they don't go smoothly, it helps to lower expectations and embrace the reality of "good enough."
- As my mother used to say: "Happiness doesn't come from having what you want, but from wanting what you have."

Good Enough
Offa's Dyke Path: Monmouth to Llanvetherine

For me a day is blessed when seven out of ten variables go our way, when my attention remains on the pleasures at hand, rather than the difficulties ahead, and when, placing one foot in front of the other, we arrive at our destination reasonably dry and just about on time. This was such a day. ❧

Taking Time
South Downs Way: Rodmel to Ditchling Beacon

On a vacation we expect to slow down. On this one I often have to. For someone as mechanically challenged as I am, just making a phone call or manipulating unfamiliar plumbing requires time I never expend at home. And I cannot do either without first putting on my glasses. Tonight, I forgot to take them with me into the shower, where a cryptic sort of operation manual was encoded on a plastic fixture. Rewrapped and partially dressed, I had to tiptoe down a cold corridor back to my room to fetch them, then return to undress and try again to extract some hot water. ❧

Slowing Down
Uphill to Old Harry: Cheddar to Wells

At home I walk about three miles an hour. I am not a speed walker. Today, however, like most days on the path, we averaged only two miles an hour because we stopped to chat, rest, and eat. As the fog seeped in, we also paused to orient ourselves, check our directions, and confirm several questionable waymarks.

At one point, three paths converged, ours and two others carved into the earth by sheep and cattle. Uncertain, we inspected the ambiguous signage and studied our map, taking time to look about until we felt confident about which of these to follow.

How lovely it is to be able to take the time we need. ❧

Up and Over
Dales Way near Buckden

I'm in my stride. In the groove. As graceful as a gazelle. But not for long. On the path ahead looms a brake on my rhythm. Another hurdle. Stile number "I don't know anymore" on this bucolic obstacle course.

There is nothing for it but to scale it. I know the drill: leg up, set pole, leg over, pole over, reset pole, step down, watch the mud. Done.

Dogs get to use the more convenient canine stile next to ours. Theirs is an easier drill: dog wags tail, dog waits, human lifts board blocking opening, dog lopes through, dog looks back to see what is taking human so long. Human lowers board, scales human stile, and catches up with dog. 🐾

Stiles are contraptions that allow humans to scale walls and fences in ways that keep livestock where it belongs. On many trails, stiles are numerous and varied. The more walls and fences there are (and there are uncounted thousands in Yorkshire), the more creative will be the opportunities for getting over them.

Stiles make every path into an exercise trail. At one station, you stop and swing your leg over. At the next, you climb a ladder. Move on a bit, and you ascend and then descend a short flight of stairs. Further on, you squeeze through a V-shaped break in a wall, after which you climb up and over a farm gate. Then you pivot around inside a circular device while moving a hinged internal gate.

This stile-sprinkled agility course is a testament to the character and ingenuity of a culture that erects a profusion of walls and then invites guests with rucksacks to scale them. Without stiles, a rambler might wither on one side of a barrier with no safe, convenient way to get over or through it.

"To count or not to count stiles?" That is the question. When we walked the Offa's Dyke Path, I gave it a go and counted every barrier I climbed over (farm gates, as well as walls) for which there was no level alternative. I did not include gates that were already open. Over a distance of some two hundred miles, our total was a stunning 433 stiles. But who's counting?

I have come to view every stile as a reminder that, eventually, we all need assistance to get beyond or through some difficulty. Each stile provides a reason to be grateful that someone we'll never know devised a structure to give us a leg up when we needed one and made it possible for us to carry on.

TIP : 11.2 A SAMPLER OF STILE STYLES

On many paths, ramblers encounter several "stile opportunities" for getting up and over obstacles. Some of the most common ones are described below.

· *Steps over walls:* Built of wood or stone. Sometimes two steps up and two down. Or one very big step up and another down because the second step has crumbled with age or was never there. Steps may be only one boot wide. A good exercise in balance.

· *Stone steps built into walls:* Never wide enough, and usually requiring an angled ascent, but sufficient to get you over a high wall.

· *Stairs and doors:* After balancing on your way up, you confront challenge number two: opening a door at the summit, squeezing yourself and your pack through, and closing it. Best negotiated when you are in the middle of a group and can avoid door-opening-and-closing responsibilities.

· *Ladders:* Variations of stairs but higher and with rungs that are even narrower than steps. You walk up facing a wall, turn yourself around at the top to face the wall again, and carefully step down backward. Easier if you hand your poles to someone else.

· *Ersatz ladders:* Better known as farm gates that won't open. You scale slippery metal or wooden slats, hoist yourself over, turn around, and, taking care not to let your pack pull you backwards, descend slowly. If you can, climb and descend a gate on the side closest to the hinges where the gate provides the most support. Try to avoid the muck at the bottom.

· *Gates:* Push open, walk through, and close. Often complicated by missing or malfunctioning hinges that require you to lift a gate, push it open (often through muck), and drop it back into place. Unlatching gates can present a challenge as well.

- *Kissing gates:* Squared off or circular, often with an internal, hinged section. Open the gate. Squeeze in. Scoot around. Close the gate, and walk out. Can be awkward if the space is skinny and your pack is fat. You may have to climb partway up the structure and shuffle around if your pack won't fit. If someone you fancy is coming in as you're going out— well, it's a kissing gate after all.

- *Skinny wall openings:* Often V-shaped, located in dry walls, and about as high as your hips. Large enough for a human to squeeze through (perhaps with some difficulty). Under-standably unpopular with the four-hoofed set.

TIP : 11.3 STILE PRINCIPLES

- Take special care when you see barbed wire across the top or along the edges of a stile. Keep yourself and your clothing from coming in contact with it.

- The best blackberries always hang over the most awkward step of a stile. Take hold of something solid before you gather them.

- Where farm gates replace stiles, leave them as you find them. When in doubt, close them.

TIP : 11.4 DISCOVERING STILES EVERY DAY

- Stiles usually appear when you need one to ease your journey.

- They will be there to lift you up, and let you down gently.

- When an obstacle blocks your path, look for someone or something to be your stile—to hold you up and assist you over hurdles.

TIME CAPSULE — COTSWOLD WAY: STANWAY

We are seated in the kitchen of the old bakehouse where we plan to spend the night. Our hostess is explaining, as she prepares our tea, that for centuries baking had been done right here for the manor house, a short distance away.

The current "Lord of the Manor," she says, is a scholar of history "at university," who lives in Stanway House with his wife and family part of the year. He still owns much of the village. The villagers pay their rents quarterly and in person, as they have done for centuries, by depositing their pounds sterling into a hole in the center of a large table located in the main hall.

We admired the elegant facade of Stanway House from the trail before arriving at its old bakehouse. Its beautifully restored tithe barn, our hostess explains as she places homemade tea cakes before us, is used today as the village hall. She believes the reason her community has maintained its historical integrity and charm is that, since the Renaissance, much of the village has belonged to a family that values and preserves tradition.

"The current lord," she says, "is Stanway's guardian and protector against the holiday cottage—the bane of many villages these days."

We sleep well in the lord's old bakehouse, in his village where, for now, time is standing still.

Sleeping Around — Cotswold Way: North Nibley

I'm getting used to occupying a different bed every night. Exercise and fresh air promote sound sleep in strange places. Still, I've been thinking about the advantages of a guided tour with a minibus that would collect us at day's end and deposit us for several consecutive nights in the same inn and a familiar bed. Some day, perhaps, Mike and I will arrange to stay at one (carefully selected) B & B for three or four nights. Our host, or a taxi, could collect us from near the trail, take us to our lodging each evening, and return us the next morning to the place where we left the path.

Some walkers choose to camp out because they can sleep inside the same sleeping bag and tent each night. This saves them the bother and expense of arranging and paying for lodging. But a camping alternative, even if it includes a well-appointed caravan, holds no appeal for a tenderfoot, who never contemplates rugged alternatives.

For now, I'm content to face another unfamiliar B & B, which, as usual, we selected from the list in our trail accommodation guide because it was close to the path, was the right distance from our last lodging, and had a vacancy when we called from the States.

Tonight we will be sleeping in North Nibley, in a grand home that looks like a set from Masterpiece Theater. It was built centuries ago and is being lovingly restored. Two of our own bedrooms back home would fit inside tonight's gigantic room, which is not at all like the room we slept in last night and won't, we are certain, resemble the one we'll sleep in tomorrow night. The space is interesting. Unique. And we are glad to be here.

After a week of walking, almost everything gets easier, as days settle into the rhythm of familiar routine. Hills seem flatter, trail maps are more decipherable, unpacking and repacking become routine, and packs rest comfortably on hips and shoulders. But nights, and their B & B adventures, remain a challenge: different beds—some soft, many softer; unique bathrooms with detailed instructions required to operate their non-standardized plumbing; electrical outlets so odd that even British guests ask for operating instructions; rooms frequently cold, rarely hot, occasionally temperate; some rooms on noisy streets, but most quiet and restful; and new hosts every night with new rules and opinions.

For tonight, however, all is well. We are clean and comfy. Our laundry is drying. Our duvet, thick and inviting, beckons.

Pleasant dreams surely will follow.

Hard Day — Uphill to Old Harry

Molasses
Cerne Abbas to Dorchester

My pack seems heavy today, my legs glued to the path. Have my boots gained weight overnight? Did Mike slip an extra water bottle or his lunch into my pack? Am I wearing less and carrying more?

What's going on? I've been prancing along for days. Why am I dragging now on this easy terrain, under a sunny sky, after a good night's sleep and a sensible English breakfast? Why do I feel weighed down like a crab under a barnacle-encrusted shell?

Hard days, it seems, just happen. Sometimes they make no sense at all, except to remind us to savor the easier ones. All we can do is trudge through their molasses, hopeful that tomorrow their mysterious burden will lift.

TIP : 11.5 HARD DAY DEFENSES
: · Hard days are random and unpredictable.
: · You just have to get through them. Form doesn't count.
: · Think of them as opportunities to practice mind over
:   matter.
: · Try not to fantasize about returning to bed or calling a taxi.
: · Hard days don't last. Press forward, count your blessings,
:   absorb your surroundings, sing a tune, and rejoice because
:   tomorrow your load will feel lighter.

Where Are We?

WAYMARKS — SOUTH DOWNS WAY

Standing in a pasture, looking for evidence of a footpath, I'm certain of only one thing. Whichever way we proceed, the soles of my boots will soon be clogged with sheep droppings.

Fog settles on our shoulders, as we watch the trail across the green expanse sink into the mist. The gate through which we entered once displayed an acorn blaze and an arrow to point our way. (We can see the telltale outline where they had been affixed.) Now, they are missing-in-action—probably removed by someone to decorate a bedroom wall or by an irate farmer whose livestock wandered through a gate left open by a careless walker. Although most waymarks remain in place, these two—crucial to our progress—have been removed.

I stare into the field, ranting at walkers' associations that refuse to sell these collectible, decorative waymark signs at visitor centers and on websites. Unavailable for purchase, they tempt every walker who wants a trail marker to remove one that's still in use. Mike and I have (so far) resisted the temptation to take one home as a souvenir because we know how much we and other walkers depend on them.

Even when acorn markers remain securely fastened to trees, fences, and barns, or are painted on stone walls, they are often not as helpful as we'd like. Many appear to have been installed arbitrarily on a sunny day by folks who already know the way and won't ever need to follow the arrows intended to guide others.

And there appears to be another reason for ambiguous signage, which becomes obvious after several wrong turns. Walkers, it seems, are expected to read guide books and consult maps and GPS units. Waymarks are considered optional. Well-placed, accurate signs would make orienteering too easy and getting lost more difficult. And what fun would that be?

We check our trail guide and peer into the gloom, relieved to see a walker approaching on what must be our path. We ask about the way ahead and soon move on with renewed confidence into the pasture and across the droppings.

Hide and Seek — South Downs Way
Meonstoke to Winchester

There are four levels of getting lost on a countryside walk, none deeply troubling. The least upsetting, Level A, occurs when you realize that either the trail or your map is not making sense. You come about, retrace your steps a bit, and look for the marker or the turn you overlooked.

This escalates to Level B when you are soaked and tired. It raises to Level C if retracing involves several extra miles of walking, the walking is uphill or through nettles and brambles, and this is your second or third wrong turn of the day. It reaches Level D when night is approaching and your blood sugar is plummeting. At Level D, good sportsmanship slips easily into orneriness, and rebellion looms.

Walkers get lost for many reasons, including questionable orienteering skills, lack of attention, and my favorite (because someone else is to blame)—an ambiguous map, confusing trail guide, or misleading waymark, like the one that was our nemesis on the final day of our South Downs Way walk, when we were victims of sabotage!

———————————————

After wandering off course an extra mile or so along a scenic old railroad bed, we arrive in a community where our luck improves. A gentleman in tweeds is working in his front yard. I suppress all cranky thoughts and inquire with a smile about the location of our missing trail.

"About two miles over that hill. Lost your way, then?"

"Right. We're not sure where we went wrong," Mike says. "But it must have been outside Meonstoke."

"You might have done. Some folks near there don't like the trail passing close by. So, when they feel like it, they remove the waymarks and send walkers, like you, in the wrong direction. We see quite a few ramblers come this way. Just follow the shortcut across that field back to your trail. You're all right now."

His reassuring conclusion is a matter of opinion. It's three o'clock, and we have six miles to go to reach Winchester, then another mile or so to our final B & B. I'm approaching Level D. My sportsmanship, however, holds.

In my tired bones, I know I'm going to make it. And I intend to enjoy every last mile that remains.

TIP : 11.6 AVOID GETTING LOST

- Ask other walkers to direct you. But check what they tell you.
- Follow waymarks, but not too literally.
- Use a compass.
- Trust your instincts.
- Consult your guide book and map frequently.
- Carry a GPS device—which we finally (and happily) did on our last three walks.

TRAIL GUIDES — OFFA'S DYKE PATH
LLANVETHERINE TO CAPEL-Y-FFIN

Robin, our British walking companion, is keeper of the *Offa's Dyke Path–National Trail Guides* (printed in two volumes, North and South), as we make our way toward Knighton. The volume he's using is protected inside a nylon case, which hangs from a long cord about his neck. The map case is an accessory sported by all properly attired, in-country ramblers.

When Robin wants to check a map or read about the path, he flips up the case and reads through its clear plastic side. I like to glance over his shoulder at the Ordnance Survey map printed in the book to inspect its converging contour lines and preview the hills ahead. Topographic lines do not lie, and when I see them bunching together, I groan.

Today, my curiosity is short-circuited. Robin raises and lowers his map before I am able to inspect its topo lines. Satisfied, he says, "No problem. Very good. Carry on."

Seeing the twinkle in his eye and the Brecon Beacons looming in the distance, I don't need a map to tell me that the way ahead is up. Then down and up again. But I am confident that, once the topo lines have been scaled, the views of green expanse will be worth every uphill step.

"Very good," I repeat. "Very good indeed."

National trail guides are the "go-to" books for planning walks on Britain's excellent national trails. You'll probably want to carry one with you to supplement strip maps or Ordnance Survey maps. Because these guides are rather heavy softcover books, it's not uncommon for ramblers to lighten their loads by tearing out and discarding the pages they no longer need.

National trail guides provide trail-specific information. They include maps, written directions, and background material on geology, history, and wildlife. They describe optional village walks and tell which services (postboxes, pubs, bike shops, farriers, and more) are available in communities. They also contain photos that will entice you to try to find the spot from which they were taken.

Unofficial trail guides that describe various walks can be useful as well. Many trail-specific guides today can be ordered on-line or through bookstores.

For lodging selection, places to dine, and general sightseeing information, however, you'll want to consult a path's accommodation guide (available for national trails, the Coast to Coast Walk, and several other routes) and a general guide book as well. It's best to do this before leaving home, so you can leave these extra books—and their extra weight—behind.

Unfortunately, trail guides are seldom convenient to carry or read, even for a walker decked out with a proper map case. This ubiquitous trekking gear, usually made from sturdy nylon, has a clear (often scratched) plastic side through which to read Ordnance Survey maps and guide books. The case is supposed to protect these paper products in wet weather, but if you need to turn a page or refold a map in the rain, wet is inevitable. In addition, the map case, on its long cord, is rather uncomfortable for foreigners, who haven't grown up walking with guide books tied to their necks.

Today, you will also see walkers wearing a second chord that disappears into a convenient pocket where a GPS unit resides. Technically advanced, these devices supplement Ordnance Survey maps, compasses, and trail guides, which many walkers, who go digital, still carry for back-up.

Occasionally, guides and maps can cause anxiety. One glance at an elevation profile of a peak, and I begin lobbying for an alternate route around it. One look at topographical lines converging at right angles to our trail, and I think about giving up before tackling the steep slope ahead. Happily, silhouettes and contours often appear more demanding than they are. The preview is almost always worse than the show.

Although imperfect, trail guides are decidedly useful. It's nice to have them handy to tell us what's ahead. They also provide helpful information both in advance and underway. So enjoy what you read, but be assured: Walking a trail is always more fun than reading a guidebook.

TIP ⋮ 11.7 GUIDELINES

⋮ · National trail guides are available for national trails in the UK. They contain selected sections, or "strips," from much larger Ordnance Survey maps, along with narrative descriptions of trails. They may be all you need to navigate a path or plan a walk. But should you need to leave a trail, the small strip maps in the trail guides may not provide sufficient information, which is why many walkers carry both a trail guide and full-sized Ordnance Survey maps. (See Step Fourteen, "Good Maps.")

⋮ · To avoid surprises, review your guide thoroughly before leaving home, and make appropriate notations wherever confusion is likely to occur.

⋮ · If you don't wish to hang a map case from your neck (and we don't), you can carry your trail guide in a convenient external pouch or in your pack. You will be consulting it frequently, so you'll want to keep it handy. A plastic bag will help keep it dry.

· Many trail associations offer their own helpful trail and accommodation guides. You can contact their offices by phone or go on-line to review and order the information they publish.

· You can obtain full-sized Ordnance Survey maps of areas you'll be visiting. But keep in mind that you may need to carry several, and maps add weight.

· The best guide we ever carried (and one I wish every trail association would emulate as an example of how to describe a trail) was as light as a feather, clear as a bell, and easy to follow. We were able to put away our national trail guide to read at night, and we never went astray. So, should you ever walk the Dales Way, order in advance (or stop in the Ilkley Tourist Center and buy) a copy of the *Dales Way Route Guide with Associated Walks* by Arthur Gemmell and Colin Speakman. It contains specially drawn maps that illustrate all the information a walker requires to stay on the trail, and it does this with clarity that is unsurpassed. It is as near to perfect as a guide gets.

SHORTCUT TEMPTATION — SOUTH DOWNS WAY
AMBERLEY TO COCKING

We are looking at a side trail that will take us up and over the hill ahead. It's not the "official" path, which leads around the rise. But taking it directly over the top will save us a mile or two. Very tempting, especially on this 11.5 mile, hard-to-dress-for day.

I've been in and out of layers all morning. Up hill, take off hat. Into the wind, cover up. After exertion, remove a layer. At a rest stop, add a layer. A dress-up/dress-down day like this one is a lot of work. So I'm considering the up/down shortcut in front of us.

By nature, I'm a committed personal energy saver, who views shortcuts as pragmatic choices, rather than as forms of cheating. For a recipe that calls for vegetable stock, I will substitute a can of organic veggie broth. Give me scissors or (oh dear!) a clipper, and I'll show you an old, well-groomed terrier who seldom sees a stripping knife.

But I do not choose the shortcut ahead. I would, if I were injured or caught out in a downpour. I would, if we had to meet someone and were running late. Certainly, I am tempted. But I will not succumb. I want to walk the South Downs Way the proper way, all the way—because I can, and because that's what I've come more than three thousand miles to do.

"Okay," I say, "Around it is. Let's go."

TIP : 11.8 SHORTCUTTING

· Lots of walkers take shortcuts.

· Shortcuts can be very helpful.

· Taking one is an acceptable option. It's not cheating. It's not a sin.

· When faced with a choice of paths, listen to your heart, and consider your own feet, the weather, and the time of day.

· Do not ask, "Which trail would others choose?" *Stepping out* means selecting the path that's best for you.

🌿 Journal

It's Worth It
Cotswold Way

We are crossing a mown field en route from Chipping Campden to Stanway. Halfway across I pose for a photo, standing next to hay bales stacked three times my height. The first full day of our one-hundred-mile walk is sunny and clear. I am starting to wonder if such glorious weather and the quaint, travel-brochure scenery are too good to last and how I'll do on the hills in the distance.

"How steep are those hills up ahead?" I ask Mike as we rest against the dry bales that loom over us.

Before he can answer, a woman seventy-five yards away, peddling her bicycle along a lane, waves and hollers, "It's worth it." I grin and wave back.

Who could ask for a more auspicious answer? 🀄

Carry on. We're almost there.

Step 12

Finishing Touches
Coming to an End

"What lies behind us and what lies before us
are tiny matters compared to what lies within us."

RALPH WALDO EMERSON
(1803–1882)

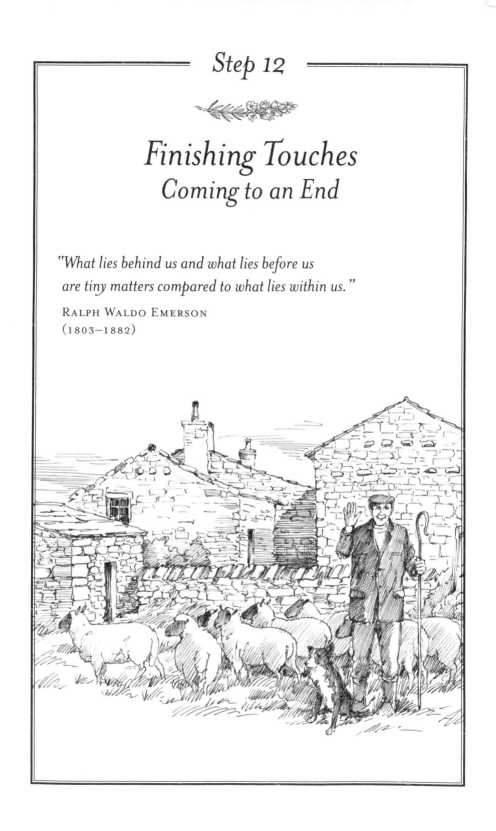

Ambivalence

Happy Endings

Lovely Lanes and Lively History

Stepping Out

Ambivalence

The final miles of a journey on foot are steps of mixed emotions. You're impatient to finish, but want to keep on walking. You can't wait to celebrate, but don't want the path to end. You're ready to shed your pack, but not ready to pick up the obligations and demands you left at home.

Then, the final waymark is before you, proclaiming the end of the path. You pose for a victory photo. You're jubilant; you're sad. You feel relieved; you feel restless. You've finished, but cannot let go. The momentum that each morning propelled you to lace up your muddy boots still impels you to step out and walk another day.

You expect to ramble again tomorrow through the countryside, wet or dry, traveling across moor and vale, your steps practiced and secure, as you move at two miles an hour along a track where mind and body connect in an adventure that fills the soul. But this is impossible. Your ramble is over. You must leave the path behind.

Near the end of a walk, thoughts and feelings tumble about like ping-pong balls in a lottery drawing. We'll explore some of these emotions as we finish our journey together, confident that we want to return to ramble again. By the time we reach our final waymark, *stepping out* will have become irresistible, and countryside walking will be a passion.

✤ J o u r n a l

A Lot of Help from My Friend
Offa's Dyke Path: Llandegla to Llangynhafal

Walking today on grassy paths, looking down on green expanses more vast than my heart can absorb, I feel anxious. Yesterday, my back began to hurt, and I'm worried that the pain will cut short our two-hundred-mile trek. With only thirty miles to go, I resent this. We have come so far. I want to finish alongside Mike, who deserves an untroubled, happy ending.

Months ago he worked for days laying out our itinerary and reserving our accommodations. Together with our British friend, Robin, he's been navigating between waymarks for almost 170 miles, carrying our extras without complaint. Even nursing a mild blister, he remains upbeat, enthusiastic, and patient.

When I whine about little things, Mike listens and assures me that they are little things. He waits patiently as I answer nature's calls and layer up or down in response to the whims of weather. Every time I wriggle into and out of my pack, he is there holding it to prevent injury to my back. He is in perpetual vacation mode: happy and "in the moment."

For Mike's sake, as well as my own, I want all that's been well to end well. I couldn't have come this far without him, without his help and encouragement, without the kindness and care of my dearest friend. ❀

❀ Journal

Homestretch
Coast to Coast Walk: Littlebeck to Robin Hood's Bay

We start out from our B & B about ten. We're not in a hurry. We want to remember our final day as a pleasant one. As we walk, my feelings are mixed. One part of me can't wait to reach Robin Hood's Bay. The other part wishes we weren't about to conclude our two-hundred-mile adventure.

Life on the trail has been simple. One pack and a two-item to-do list: wash laundry, write post cards. No meals to plan, no errands to run, no phone calls or e-mails to answer. Our worries have been reduced to the basics: health, weather, and finding our way. Nothing else has mattered.

I grow restless and nervous as we approach the end. I'm excited about reaching a goal that means almost too much. I'm anxious to be done with something I didn't think I could do, but I also want to keep on walking.

Caution is starting to consume me, and I take great care to place my feet securely. I don't want to stumble or turn an ankle now.

Outside the fishing village of Robin Hood's Bay we rest on a bench overlooking the sea and our destination, hard-by the rocky shore below. I want to dance, but restrain myself—premature celebration might tempt fate. Instead, tears fill my eyes as reality seeps in. Happiness fills my heart and travels out my limbs. We really are going to do this!

We put on our packs one last time, for two more miles, and ramble on. ❀

Stones for Offa
Offa's Dyke Path: Prestatyn

For much of the day we've been treated to distant views of Prestatyn, the seaside community where our journey will end. Robin, Mike, and I finally arrive there in late afternoon after a cliffside walk and a series of very steep hills—the final challenges for strengthened, but weary, muscles. Passing a fenced yard, we are startled by angry sounds of crashing and snarling. A gigantic bull mastiff peers down at us from the top of a wooden barrier, against which he is hurling his massive bulk. We pick up our pace, tired muscles forgotten. The triumphant last mile of a ramble is no time to fend off an attacking canine.

At our B & B we chat with our hosts while we relax over iced tea and Scottish shortbread in the afternoon sun, savoring the satisfaction of a fine finish. At last we are ready. We leave our packs behind in our cheerful rooms and set out to honor an Offa's Dyke tradition.

It is a mile through the tidy town to the beach where we snap pictures beneath the final waymark set at the northern end of the path. Then we move onto the sand where each of us removes a small stone from a pocket. We collected these at the southern end of the trail in Chepstow. They have traveled with us for more than 195 miles. We'd like to carry them home. But tradition demands otherwise.

We step to the water's edge. And one by one, with gratitude in our hearts, we fling our stones into the Irish Sea to bid King Offa adieu. ❧

Crowing
Offa's Dyke Path: Prestatyn

The woman who cast her stone upon the waters of the Irish Sea has grown whole and strong. She can live for three weeks out of a pack she can carry on her back. She is able to move beyond the familiar. For two hundred miles she got through, made do, carried on, stayed focused, lived in the present, tolerated discomfort (with some whining), and accepted most of the arbitrary rules set by a culture she has come to love.

I don't recognize her yet. But she's someone I am getting to know. ❧

RAMBLER'S REWARDS

You don't need to complete an entire journey to luxuriate in satisfaction.
It's the gift a walker opens at the conclusion of every day.

Each evening, after I master the plumbing, and shower or soak in a bath, I dress in my cleaner clothes. I sip hot tea (hopefully in a warm room) while my hair dries, and our laundry hangs from a line or lies draped over a radiator. Muscles and bones relax. Contentment settles in. Conversation is easy and agreeable.

This is a pleasant time for anticipating the evening ahead: a British ale, congenial meal (at which we'll indulge ourselves in whatever we fancy on the menu), and a night of sound sleep tucked under a thick comforter.

In these quiet moments, it occurs to me that, having achieved this, maybe—just maybe—I can do whatever I dream.

HUMBLE PIE — COTSWOLD WAY: BATH

☙ J o u r n a l

Invisible

Our first view of Bath at the end of the Cotswold Way is stunning. We look down on golden limestone architecture from a high point framed in blue flowers that in a few weeks will be magically transformed into capsules full of tiny flax seeds.

Soon we are walking among shoppers and "holiday makers" on a pedestrian mall, approaching Bath's famous Pump Room. I wonder if these strangers can see our joy or sense our feelings of accomplishment. Do they even notice the graying couple carrying full packs? 🦙

Not likely. Walkers are a common sight in this nation of avid ramblers. Completing a one-hundred-mile trek, although something worth celebrating and a reason to feel proud, is not a remarkable accomplishment here. Which is why, upon entering Bath, I feel satisfied, relieved, and happy, but not especially impressed with myself.

Perhaps, at last, I have become a walker. And walkers know that they control and can take credit for just a small portion of a journey's outcome.

Everything else—health, weather, good accommodations—are mostly a matter of luck.

Even in my euphoria at the end of a trail, I'm aware that I did not create my own success. Nor did I scale Mt. Everest—although at times I might have thought I had. I simply went on a countryside walk and had the good fortune to reach its end in fine health, having had enough time along the way to savor its daily delights and fill my senses with small villages and grand vistas; with bilberries, blackberries, and elderberries; with wood pigeons, rooks, and ravens; with sloe, plums, and figs; with mountain ash and high-bush cranberry; with heather, thistle, and ivy-carpeted woodland; and with the scents of flowers and the peace of quiet places.

NOSTALGIA

At the conclusion of every walk, we begin thinking about our next ramble, when we will once again return to the daily routines of a footpath, to landscapes that captivate us, and to full English breakfasts. We think about villages and farms, and the sounds, scents, and scenery that together define the British countryside. And we recall the local characters we are leaving behind.

I feel nostalgic when I think about these quirky folks, these appealing souls who raise eccentricity to an art form, these inflexible, sometimes infuriating, always fascinating, wise and witty, outspoken beings who keep drawing us back:

- A guest at our B & B in Glaisdale (Coast to Coast Walk), who has been a member of the Women's Cricket Association for sixty years and is still passionate about her sport.
- The blind sexton of a Methodist chapel in Littlebeck (near the end of our Coast to Coast Walk), who bid us a safe arrival home and that we "find everything there as we wished it to be." Kindness is so comforting.
- A cyclist named Bob, a guest at our B & B in Capel-y-ffin (Offa's Dyke Path), who rides between the hedges along narrow roads in Wales for hundreds of miles, rain or shine, most weekends and every vacation, on a bike he assembled that seems to have everything a seventy-five-year-old aficionado would want.

- Our host at a B & B in Danby Wiske (Coast to Coast Walk) who told me at breakfast (which was served in his unheated dining room) that "being warm is a state of mind" and that "if you tell yourself you're warm, you'll feel comfortable." Trapped in a fifty-five degree room, I was not about to argue. As I hurried through breakfast, I tried thinking heated thoughts, but never did warm up.
- Walkers we met, who said that our packs looked "sensible," and that our itinerary and slow rate of travel was "very nice." "It gives you time," they observed, "to look about and enjoy the countryside, doesn't it?" Encouragement and acceptance mean so much.
- The Yorkshire farmer, dressed in "working tweeds," repairing a tractor on a rainy morning, who watched us coming up the path encased in rain gear and said without a trace of sarcasm, "Great day, isn't it?" His cheerfulness was contagious and transformed our wet morning into a fine day.
- Many other colorful folks who know, and are prepared to tell a visitor, what is "proper." And who never stop being themselves.

Their faces, their idiosyncrasies, are stored in our memories. We exercise our smile muscles just thinking about them. As we board a train or bus on the first leg of our return journey to the States, we take them with us. And we always wonder: Are we leaving or returning home?

Happy Endings

Enticing Finales

Each walk offers its own, unique conclusion. Some end with special traditions. Many invite us to explore the community in which a trail ends or another interesting area close by. Below are some post-ramble locations we've enjoyed visiting before traveling back to the States.

Winchester (end of the South Downs Way)

Since the twelfth century, weary travelers have been stopping at St. Cross Hospital in Winchester to receive the wayfarer's dole—a loaf of bread and cup of ale. So, after a night of rest and in keeping with this tradition marking the end of a journey, we approach the hospital to ask for "the dole." A porter in the gatehouse offers us a small biscuit (cookie) and a tumbler of ale, tokens of those earlier offerings.

We purchase two small dole cups thrown by a local potter. They are replicas of a larger one of medieval vintage that the gatekeeper invites us to inspect. His has been carved from a horse's hoof and is set into a silver holder. We look forward to filling our own modest cups with a stout or porter a few days from now, when we toast the South Downs Way from across the Atlantic.

St. Cross Hospital is Britain's oldest charitable institution. We visit its public rooms and church, which take us back to the days of knights and sandal-footed wayfarers. The remainder of the day we walk about Winchester, which was inhabited by both Britons and Romans before the Anglo-Saxons made it the capital of their Kingdom of Wessex, beginning in about 495 and ending with the death of King Alfred in 899.

After the Norman conquest, Winchester remained one of England's centers of learning and commerce. With its famous cathedral, old Norman castle, public school, and historic sights, this comfortable town, often overlooked by tourists, appears relatively untouched by modern construction and industry. It is an attractive, genuine step back into history, and we wish we had more than one day to explore.

Windermere (end of the Dales Way)

This vacation community is located in the heart of the Lake District, a beautiful region of mountains and lakes about thirty miles long and twenty miles wide in northwestern England. The Lake District has been a favorite haunt for artists and writers, including such notables as William Wordsworth, Samuel Taylor Coleridge, Robert Southey, and Beatrix Potter.

In Windermere, you can enjoy a cruise aboard an elegant Edwardian steamboat on the largest lake in the region, walk through this charming tourist town where tea shops and cafes abound, visit the Lake District National Park Visitor Centre, or hop aboard a minibus for a sightseeing/cultural tour of the area. We did all four in one day with time to spare for me to attend a Rotary Club dinner meeting.

We departed from Windermere on the Settle-to-Carlisle scenic railway, which took us back through much of the countryside we had seen on foot, providing one last, glorious gaze at the Dales—an encore through a train window—and a perfect finish.

Whitby (end of the Coast to Coast Walk)

The night we completed our C-to-C walk we stayed at a B & B in Robin Hood's Bay. The next morning we took a public bus to Whitby, less than a half-hour away. Whitby is a perfect post-ramble haven, mostly undiscovered by Americans. It is easy to explore and a "just-right" finale for the C-to-C walker.

Once an old fishing village, the town is a mecca for British "holiday makers" and the home of Whitby jet, an elegant black stone used in jewelry and other crafts. Charming and picturesque, Whitby's history includes such illustrious names as Queen Boudicca, who led a rebellion against the Romans (61 AD), and Captain James Cook, who, among his many seafaring adventures, circumnavigated the globe (1771). Today, this former whaling port, which is featured in Bram Stoker's Dracula, invites visitors to stroll its historic streets and enjoy its restaurants and comfortable accommodations.

Bath (end of the Cotswold Way)

At the south end of the Cotswold Way is the remarkable city of Bath. Just ninety minutes by train from London, it is a "must see" UNESCO World Heritage Site. Infused with elegant, cream-colored Georgian architecture, Bath has been attracting tourists since the Romans discovered its hot waters and built their famous baths here.

The city is handsome and a delight to visit on foot. With its two excellent museums, five-hundred-year-old abbey, stately Royal Crescent, and charming canal boats (moored a short distance from the center of town), Bath is an ideal city to explore and a grand place to celebrate a walk well done.

Winding Down: London

We're back! We arrive at our small hotel near Victoria station in early afternoon. Smiling staff welcome us back from our countryside adventure, handing us the duffel bag we left in hotel storage. It was from here that we set off twenty days ago, packs on our backs, to walk the two-hundred-mile Offa's Dyke Path. Now we have returned to spend our final nights in comfortable, familiar surroundings.

I take a lovely, long shower, wrap in a large, soft towel, use the hair dryer provided, and dress in the clean clothes I left behind in our duffel. We feel pampered in our well-appointed quarters: tea, biscuits (chocolate, no less!), a full set of towels for each of us (including a flannel), bedside reading lamps, a working television, an empty closet and bureau, and plenty of hooks for hanging everything.

For two nights this will be home—only better. It's more like a pause in paradise, a sojourn in a comfort zone, where one can relax between a walk well done and a busy life just a flight away.

In this middle zone, however, danger lurks. We are hungry all the time.

Tomorrow we may walk around Cambridge, Greenwich, or Trafalgar Square. But these local rambles will be less than ten miles long, and will be executed without either the calorie-burning rucksacks we've been carrying for weeks or the hilly topography to which our metabolic set-points have become accustomed. The days of "whatever we want to eat" are over.

We're calorically decompressing, but not fast enough to prevent craving and snacking. We've been trying to "just say no" to full English breakfasts and generous restaurant dinners. And we've concluded that it would be easier to put on our backpacks and head north for another two-hundred-mile ramble. ❧

Souvenirs: Heathrow Airport

Trapped in the passenger holding area beyond security check-in, I stock up on a large bag of Blend 49 tea from Harrods and fifteen rolls (a year's supply) of Trebor "extra strong" mints, powerful enough to take my breath away. With two hours before our flight, I'm doing what travelers do best— sitting and waiting. I'm also thinking about the people who recently touched our lives and daydreaming about their countryside, now as familiar to me as my own neighborhood.

In my on-flight luggage is a sand-cast figurine of a badger that I bought in Reeth and carried in my pack for a hundred miles. Also tucked away is a set of dragonfly earrings, inlaid with local black stone from Whitby, purchased on our post-ramble day at leisure. In my memory, however, I carry more: busy towns, musty bookstores, and greengrocers; cozy villages, chocolate shops, and friendly pubs; landscapes reminiscent of countryside scenes in classic hunting prints; hills and velvety dales, mountains and flowing becks, gray stone walls and kissing gates; sheep and cattle, pastures and fields; canals and castles, cities and sea coasts; hand-pumped ales and jacket potatoes; chocolate biscuits and spotted dick puddings; sights, scents, and impressions so rich and satisfying that I expect I'll feel full until I return to replenish my tea, my mints, and my memories. ❦

Lovely Lanes and Lively History

WHERE SHALL WE WANDER?

Eventually, every walker discovers a favorite walk, or perhaps several favorites. Our British rambles hold a special place in my own memory, as do a number of other walks outside of Great Britain:

• a trek in the hills of the ancient Buddhist Kingdom of Bhutan
• a walk on a section of the Inca Trail, just beyond Machu Pichu in Peru, where travelers have walked for centuries
• a day hike above Lake Wanaka on the South Island of New Zealand
    · ˙t to the lush Dordogne Valley of France where prehistoric people

once roamed and medieval hilltop villages now welcome visitors
· walks in our local, lakeside park

Perhaps, some day soon, a walk in the British countryside will find a place on your own list of favorites.

OUT OF THE PAST

Wherever I walk in Britain, I fall in love with its history and rural landscape. I may be thinking about today's weather, the late hour, or the distance ahead. I may be focused on where I need to place my feet. But what I am feeling is the pulse of the past and the presence of long-gone strangers: wayfarers, sheep herders, monks, and common folk on their way to medieval market towns. These hubs—which are often B & B locations today—were rarely more than seven or eight miles apart, because yesterday's "shoppers" were able walk that far in a morning and still have time to buy and sell their goods, break bread with neighbors, and return home at day's end.

A countryside walker follows in their footsteps and in those of other strangers: ancients, traveling in footwear of straw; Roman soldiers, marching in battle gear; friars, walking between monasteries; refugees, fleeing conquerors; pilgrims, seeking sanctuary; and ramblers and tourists, who passed this way only yesterday. These are their paths. This is their history. They walk with us as we tramp their ancient ways, moving as they did. One foot in front of the other, back through time.

Stepping Out

Well, we've made it. We're at the end of our journey together. Time to kick off our boots and wiggle our toes. Time to bask in the glow of arriving at our final waymark in good spirits. Time to celebrate the joys of unhurried, daily travel on our own two feet. Time to think back on weeks of healthful exercise and miles of conversation, on days of tiny flowers and wide expanses, on moments of grumbling and rain, laughter and sunshine.

Over the miles, we've fallen in love with walking. Already, we miss the footpaths, the people, the communities, the countryside.

We've developed a kinship with our fellow ramblers and with the ancient ones, whose spirits walked with us along canal towpaths, abandoned railways, village lanes, cliffsides, drovers' tracks, woodland paths, and remote sheep walks. We feel closer now to nature, aware of our role in sustaining its breadth and diversity, wishing we had lovely, long-distance, public footpaths through countryside closer to home.

On our gentle journey together—walking, trekking, tramping, rambling—we've been *stepping out* into new, sometimes uncomfortable, experiences, discovering strength, joy, wholeness, and peace. And hasn't it been fun!

Thank you for making the journey with me. May we meet again along the way.

Step 13

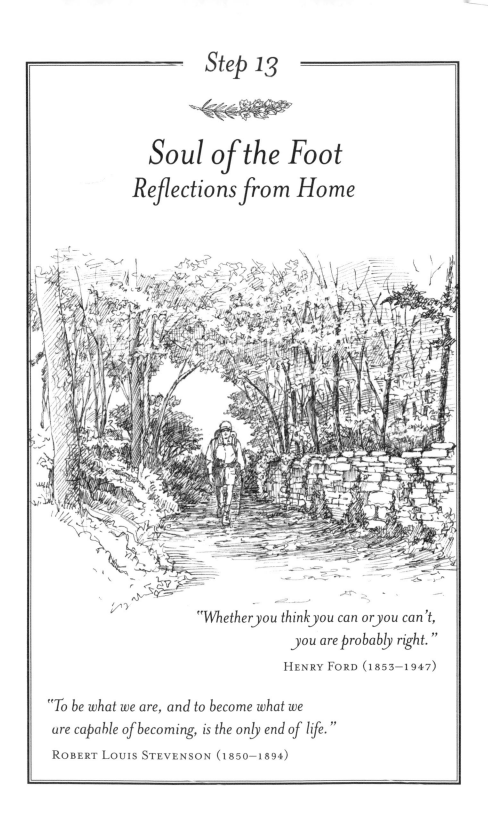

Soul of the Foot
Reflections from Home

*"Whether you think you can or you can't,
you are probably right."*

HENRY FORD (1853–1947)

*"To be what we are, and to become what we
are capable of becoming, is the only end of life."*

ROBERT LOUIS STEVENSON (1850–1894)

From the Home Front
    Tip 13.1: Settling In

Mentors and Friends

Talking the Walk

Little Lessons

Quitting

Gentle Living
    Journal: Aftereffects
    Tip 13.2: Living Like a Walker

A Walker's Wish

From the Home Front

At the end of every vacation, Mike and I arrive home to a stack of neglected demands, a consequence of forsaking daily routine for travel. Even when we return on time, in good health, and find our home undamaged, our loved ones well, and our key where the young neighbor who collects our mail is supposed to leave it, we feel dragged down by piles of "have tos" and waves of homecoming hassles that threaten to drown our post-vacation elation.

But after trekking over one hundred miles, I feel less daunted by the usual flood of obligations. Strengthened and refreshed by weeks of rambling, I stand ready to confront: two cartons filled with mail and catalogs, scores of e-mail messages (no matter that before I left home I asked friends to cease and desist), piles of laundry, an empty refrigerator, a duffel bag to unpack, and gear to stow for another ramble.

It may take a while, but, having completed a long countryside walk, I feel confident that I'll also make it to the end of my lists. And while I'm checking things off, I'll be operating familiar plumbing and sleeping in the same bed every night. How hard can that be?

TIP : 13.1 SETTLING IN

- It takes about one day per time zone before you sleep soundly again and your bodily functions return to normal. For example, if you live on the East Coast, a trip to Europe requires about five or six days of adjustment.

- Catching up—shrinking a "to-do" list down to where it was before you left home—takes about a week for every week you're away.

- After a countryside walk, lists may seem shorter because you move through them with more pep and vigor.

- *Stepping out* of who you were into the person you are now, you may be tempted, as you settle into your routine, to reconsider who it is you wish to become.

Mentors and Friends

Bob and JoAnne were our mentors for our first ramble. They had just walked the Cotswold Way, which, for us, qualified them as "experts." We took every word they uttered to heart. What they advised, we did. So, when we arrived home after our first countryside walk along the South Downs Way, we were looking forward to giving them something useful in return for their valuable advice and encouragement.

I decided to visit them on my foray into town to restock our empty refrigerator. I wanted to check on our mentors' current travel preparations. In five days they would be off on another walk, and I was certain they'd want to take with them the package of lamb's wool I was carrying in my pocket.

Handing them my small, featherweight present, I explain how wrapping and felting small strips of wool around sensitive toes can prevent and cushion blisters. An "expert" now myself, I present the wool as a gift from two new ramblers who have "been there, done that," and who plan to ramble again, blister-free.

Walkers like the four of us, regardless of experience, age, or ethnicity, regardless of political party or country of origin, happily share more than cures for blisters. We share an enthusiasm for moving slowly on foot, away from the noise and bustle of the modern world, free from contrived entertainment and the schedules and routines that dominate our lives. We prefer to walk on beaten paths, tramped by generations of travelers. We ramble in far-off lands when we can, and along local roads and paths when we cannot. We walk to restore our strength, confidence, and sense of wonder. We walk because it's fun.

For us, *stepping out* is an exploration of ourselves and our limits, a path to new experiences, a way to make friends, and a means to uncover the happiness stored beneath the "hurries" of daily living.

Talking the Walk

"I'd like to make a donation in gratitude for Mike's and my safe return from another wonderful walk in England." I'm on my feet, addressing the weekly gathering of my Rotary Club. As soon as I take my seat, the questions at my table begin. They are the same ones I've been answering since we returned and began checking in with friends and family.

Q: How far did you walk?

A: About two hundred miles.

Q: How many miles did you cover each day?

A: We averaged around eleven, which is a rate of about two miles per hour with stops.

Q: How was the weather?

A: Better than we expected, or dared to hope for—only two mornings of light rain.

Q: Where did you stay on your walk?

A: Mostly at bed and breakfasts. Sometimes at inns, youth hostels, or pubs. No camping. Nothing rugged. We make all of our reservations from the U.S. before we leave.

Q: What do you do about luggage?

A: We carry what we need on our backs. We leave what we don't want to carry at the hotel where we stay our first and last nights. Our packs weigh less than twenty-five pounds. We could hire a luggage service, but find it easier and more convenient to carry our own things.

So much for basic questions. On to other, more difficult, ones.

Q: Was your walk fun?

A: Most of the time, yes. Occasionally, no. Often, even better than fun. More like joy. A countryside walk is a journey of vivid awareness and consuming fascination, a celebration of living, moving, and growing, something utterly splendid.

Q: Why not walk here? Why go all the way to Europe?

A: Here? Where might we find open, timeless, protected landscapes and miles of public footpaths far from sprawl? Where might we discover the welcoming charm of pedestrian-friendly villages and the convenience of clean, well-run, overnight accommodations every ten miles or so?

Q: Is it hard to walk two hundred miles?

A: Not if you like to walk and do so on most days at home. A countryside walk is not a hike in the wilderness. Neither is it a scramble up a rocky mountain trail. It is a modest trek, a mild tramp, a pleasant ramble with friends. It is what humans were designed to do. It is sensible and completely natural. You do it to enjoy it—no matter how far you walk.

Q: Where did you walk?

A: We walked in Britain on paths protected and preserved by today's ramblers for those who will follow in their footsteps. There are hundreds of off-road trails across thousands of miles of countryside. Many cross private property and wend through remote forests, active farms, and pleasant villages as they have done for centuries.

Q: Will you be doing this again?

A: We hope so. Health, wealth, and time permitting, we'd love to take another "walk on the mild side." The truth is, we would have a hard time staying away from long-distance walking, hooked as we are on encounters with engaging characters and the exploration of scenic footpaths through working landscapes and charming communities.

Little Lessons

I'm packing away my gear and clothing, hoping I'll remember where I placed these things the next time I need them. Along with my rambling duds, I'm also tucking away some lessons I learned on our walk, adding them to other lessons collected on other walks. I will try to remember them as I go about my daily tasks. Like dry, warm clothing on a cold, wet day, wisdom gained from *stepping out* comforts, sustains, and reassures.

• Lesson One: *Life is like a funnel.*
 If you push through the narrow end and do difficult things first, whatever follows will be easier. This is why a high hill makes the peaks in the distance less daunting and why a trek of one hundred miles makes daily walking back home a breeze—no matter what the weather.

- Lesson Two: *Courage is relative.*

If a challenge seems difficult or frightening, and you do it anyway—in spite of dread and in defiance of reluctance—you are committing an act of courage. You don't need to climb Mt. Everest to exhibit bravery. You only need to do something that makes you uneasy—like fording a stream by teetering on slippery rocks when your balance is a bit off, and you have no choice because your path crosses the beck. So you "give it a go." In the rain. Carrying your pack. Brilliant.

- Lesson Three: *Our imperfect bodies are more capable than we think.*

If you are blessed with a body that works reasonably well, you can take a countryside walk—in spite of aches, pains, allergies, assorted complaints, and chronic reminders of age and disuse. Tramping is a physical and emotional stretch that feels terrific.

- Lesson Four: *Moving beyond one's comfort zone builds strength and fortitude.*

This is why we feel more confident when we push our bodies a little further, a little higher, and for a little longer than they want to go. It is also why we feel ready to meet new challenges and follow new paths after a long-distance walk.

- Lesson Five: *For a tenderfoot, experience is the mother of confidence.*
  - Once you sleep in an unfamiliar bed almost every night for several weeks, you can sleep almost anywhere.
  - Once you walk ten miles in a day, you can picture yourself walking that many miles every day for several days—or weeks.
  - Once you walk with a pack, you think about shedding possessions you thought you needed and could not live without. You may also discover that having less to carry in life makes you happy.
  - Once you move forward in a soaking rain, you know you have become a good sport. You're proud that you can tolerate discomfort. You smile more and whine less. But, being a tenderfoot, you always try your best to stay dry.
  - Once you walk one or two-hundred-miles, watch out. There will be no living with the intrepid butterfly that emerges as you spread your wings.

- Lesson Six: *"What if?" is a good question, but not a good excuse.*
  There's nothing wrong with being cautious and weighing consequences, but sometimes it's more productive—and more fun—to say, "What the hell. Let's do it." And to deal with the challenges (if they occur) later.

- Lesson Seven: *Time spent worrying is often wasted.*

  Anxiety makes things appear worse than they are. Hills look higher, distances longer, and B & Bs shabbier than they usually turn out to be. In fact, the saddest-looking, down-on-its-luck, mucky farmstead, which I worried about from the moment it came into view, turned out to be the coziest, cleanest, and most welcoming haven of an entire walk.

- Lesson Eight: *Multitasking is a habit worth breaking.*

  By remaining alert to irregularities on the footpath, the next waymark, or the location of your B & B, you'll be as absorbed as a dog on a hunt. With your senses focused and your mind engaged in walking, you'll feel liberated and invigorated. On a ramble, "single-tasking" becomes addicting—and something you'll want to try again at home.

- Lesson Nine: *Local flavor is the spice of life.*

  Add interest to your walk by talking and traveling with other ramblers (and their dogs) along a footpath. It's a great way to make new friends. Their companionship, insight, and support will enhance a ramble, bring the countryside to life, and make you think about connecting with some of the local characters in your own neighborhood.

- Lesson Ten: *The "proper way" is fine, but your own way is better.*
  Listen to your heart, and trust your intuition to tell you what to wear, how much to carry, and how far to walk. Your ramble, like your life, is your own journey. Find your own way to walk it. Choose the best path for you. *Stepping out* is a pleasure when the path you follow is your own.

Quitting

Quitting is not failing. It is simply a conclusion we reach after assessing our options. It is the decision we make when the path we're on is not the right one.

When I was in the third grade, my classmates and I planted little seeds in little pots. Under the watchful eyes of Miss Jagger and a strong light, our seeds grew into little plants, which we took home.

I placed mine on a window sill and waited for flowers like the ones on the seed package to appear. They never did. My plant's stem thickened. Its leaves broadened. But that was all. I watched and fed and watered. Nothing changed until my plant shriveled, turned yellow, and drooped. Still, I watered and watched. I wasn't giving up. I believed in the "miracle of added effort."

My mother suggested that we purchase a new plant, one with flowers already in bloom.

"No," I said. "I want this one to grow flowers."

"Well," said my mother, who knew about such things, "I don't think your plant wants to grow flowers. Perhaps it's time to let it go and to choose another."

"I'm not giving up," I insisted.

"I didn't say you were," she replied. "I said it might be time to let go of something that isn't working for you. It might be time [and here I'm translating liberally from the Yiddish] to stop hitting your head against a wall."

Why, then, when something isn't working for us, are we reluctant to abandon it? Why do we keep hitting our heads against walls, persisting when we ought to fold our proverbial cards and walk away from the table? Perhaps because we're stubborn. Perhaps because we don't know when something is inappropriate for us. Or, perhaps, because someone once told us that "giving up is failing," that "quitting is for sissies." And we believed them.

So, here and now, I'm giving every tenderfoot who starts a walk permission—in honor of my mother—to abandon part, or all, of the walk. Perhaps, walking for just one day or along one section of a footpath will be enough.

Do this if the weather is terrible, if you feel miserable, or if you're not well. Do this if you're too tired, the trail is too muddy, or the distance too great. If you've truly had it, leave the path. Quit. Change your plans. Get a ride into town or to your B & B. Dry off, rest up, and then decide what you'll do tomorrow. Give yourself permission to change your plans.

Don't feel guilty. Quitting is not giving up. It is letting go of something that isn't suitable, something that isn't meant to be. Where is it written that we have to finish everything we start, that we have to work at things that aren't working for us? Where is it written that we should keep watching and watering wilted plants and missing all the flowers?

That said, most walkers usually prefer to persevere, to go the distance and scramble over rough terrain in unpleasant conditions. Sometimes, however, they can't. When it's just too much for body and soul, when it's just not fun anymore, even determined ramblers alter plans.

Our friends, Bob and JoAnne, did this when they confronted a freak spring snowfall that choked the trail and turned their ramble into a cold, wet slog through knee-deep snow drifts. They abandoned their Cotswold Way walk and completed their holiday visiting other places in England. They quit—and returned a few years later to try again. The second time they walked the entire way in sunshine, welcomed by spring blossoms and pastel landscapes. Theirs was a good decision.

So, please, repeat after me: "Quitting isn't a crime. It's putting aside whatever isn't working for me right now. Tomorrow, things may be different. I may be different. I'll just wait and see."

Gentle Living

================================ ❧ J o u r n a l ═══

Aftereffects

Here at home my daily routines haven't changed much. But I have. Long lists of commitments don't produce the stress they once did. In spite of expanding demands, I feel as happy as a puppy on an outing. Countryside calm has followed me home.

After weeks of gentle walking, far from the demands and clamor of daily life, my perceptions and reactions have shifted. The act of moving big muscles and drawing in deep breaths on trails that stretched to the horizon has changed the ways I perceive obligations, set priorities, and measure time and distance. I still move efficiently, but at a slower speed. My senses are sharper and my connection to the natural world deeper and more meaningful as I travel a new path of gentle living. 🖎

TIP : 13.2 LIVING LIKE A WALKER

- Lighten your pack of obligations.

- Leave behind what you no longer wish to carry.

- Do one thing at a time. Give "single-tasking" a chance to become a habit.

- Divide long distances and big projects into comfortable segments.

- Ignore diversions that prevent you from reaching your destination.

- Decide which demands can wait, and let them wait. Correspondence can wait. Blisters cannot.

- Limit your worrying to things you can do something about, like watching where you place your feet and caring for your health.

- Expect occasional discomfort and difficulty. Every path has its puddles.

- Remember that life is a journey, and "smooth" is not its natural condition.

- Ignore light showers, and press on. Torrential rain is another matter. You have to deal with downpours.

- Find a new path if the one you're on leads in the wrong direction.

- Walk often. Sprint only when necessary.

- Whine if you must, but be brief.

- Absorb beauty and goodness.

- Observe details.

- Meet challenges with optimism.

- Stretch often.

- Lift carefully.

- Nourish body, soul, and mind.

- Make time for the things that make you smile—for beautiful moments and loved ones who share your journey.

A Walker's Wish

As we travel, may we be warm and well. May we walk on a path without pain. May we find joy in our accomplishments and friends to walk with us. And when the weather turns foul, may we make our way without slipping, find strength to savor the journey, and arrive at a place that is cozy and dry. *Happy Walking.*

What you are is what you have been.
What you will be is what you do now.

THE BUDDHA (C. 563–483 BCE)

Step 14

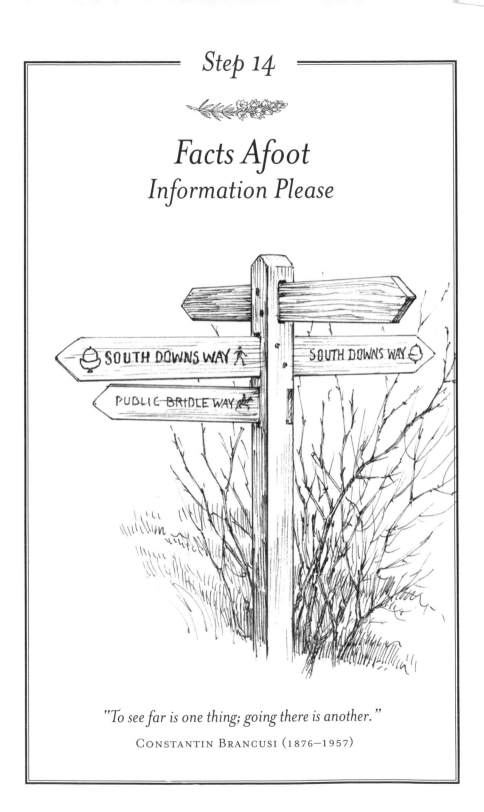

Facts Afoot
Information Please

"To see far is one thing; going there is another."

CONSTANTIN BRANCUSI (1876–1957)

Disclaimer

Starting Out: Finding Basic Information
    Tip 14.1: Dialing Telephone Numbers in the UK

Tourist Information

Cultural Sites

Walking Information

Public Transportation

Guidebooks

General Reading

Good Maps

Paths Taken

Coast to Coast Walk

Cotswold Way

Dales Way

Offa's Dyke Path

Ridgeway

South Downs Way

Uphill to Old Harry

Frequently Asked Questions

Do You Have a Favorite Path?

Are There Many Paths for Walking?

When Is the Best Time of Year to Walk?

What Is a Good Distance for a Ramble?

Is Luggage Transfer Available?

Have You Taken a Walking Tour?

What Are Your Favorite Fabrics and Items of Clothing?

Where Do You Shop?

Why Are Walking Vacations So Popular?

Do You Regret Losing Time When Stopping along a Path?

Afterthought: Step Out

Step Fourteen answers questions I'm frequently asked about the places, products, and services I particularly like. I'm rather reluctant to address such questions because my replies could be taken as recommendations, which they are not. Therefore, to avoid misunderstanding, I offer below something that has become very popular of late—a disclaimer.

Disclaimer
For Products and Services Reviewed in This Chapter

- Products mentioned here are my personal favorites as I write these pages. By the time you read them, my preferences may have changed.
- Before every walk, I discover new and improved products and replace many old favorites on my list.
- My choices are only one person's "cup of tea"—mine—and may not be suitable for you.
- Follow your own path. Shop where and how you prefer.
- The name on a label is not as important as a product's fit, comfort, durability, and function.
- Every week new companies seem to emerge, and old ones disappear. New websites appear, and familiar ones vanish. Today's preferences may be unavailable tomorrow.
- The internet is a treasure trove of assistance, but it can become overwhelming. I tend to return to a few websites that I find useful. No doubt you will discover your own favorites. Just take care that you don't drown your enthusiasm and confidence in a tsunami of information.
- Resources and references in Step Fourteen are listed in alphabetical order, not in order of personal preference.

Starting Out: Finding Basic Information

Below are my favorite first stops on the research highway. You can phone, write, or go on-line to "visit" these sources.

TIP : 14.1 DIALING TELEPHONE NUMBERS IN THE UK

• From the States, dial the international code 011, followed by the UK country code 44, then the area code and local number. Omit the first zero, if there is one. For example, if the number listed is 01234-5678, dial 011-44-1234-5678 from the States.

• In the UK dial the full number: 01234-5678. Omit the area code (ask which numbers these are) when making a local call. Note: Phone numbers in the UK do not all have the same number of digits as ours do in the States.

TOURIST INFORMATION

Tourist Information Centers (TIC) in the UK—With over 800 of these visitor oases, most towns will have one. You won't leave a TIC empty-handed. Look for maps and brochures. Find and book accommodations, tours, and more. In London you can stop by or call the Britain and London Visitors Center, 1 Regent Street, London SW1Y 4XT (020-8846-9000) during normal business hours.

Visit Britain—Formerly the British Tourist Authority (BTA), Visit Britain has offices around the world and in several U.S. cities, including an office in New York City at 551 Fifth Avenue (at 45th Street), Suite 701, New York, NY 10176-0799 (800-462-2748 or 212-986-1188; www.visit-britain.com). Ask for maps and information on walking. These materials will be mostly general in nature.

CULTURAL SITES

Many of Britain's best sites are operated by charitable organizations. If you're walking by one of these sites, you'll want to take the time to visit. The following contact information may be useful.

English Heritage is a government agency charged with promoting and protecting England's historic heritage, including many popular destinations (0870-333-1181; www.english-heritage.org.uk).

National Trust is a charity, independent of the government, that works to protect and preserve the coastline, countryside, and historic buildings of England, Wales, and Northern Ireland (0870-458-4000; www.nationaltrust.org.uk).

www.history.uk.com is a visitor-friendly website designed to help people of all ages uncover British history. Teachers and tourists alike will find answers to their questions on this website and its links. This is an excellent first stop before setting off to see historic sites.

Walking Information

Best Walks Britain lists accommodations, books on walking, maps, gear, and companies that offer guided and self-guided walking holidays (www.bestwalks.com).

National Trails is a useful, government-supported website describing fifteen national trails in England and Wales. Type in the name of a trail and receive information, enhanced with beautiful photos, to help you plan your walk and locate accommodations on national trails (www.nationaltrail.co.uk).

Natural England was established by the government to conserve and enhance England's countryside, promote access and recreation, protect landscapes and wildlife, and encourage the public's enjoyment of these priceless assets. The agency provides information about permissive access and rights-of-way (www.naturalengland.org.uk).

Ramblers' Association is Britain's largest walking organization. You'll find brochures, information on walking and accommodations, and excellent books and maps. Second Floor, Camelford House, 87-90 Albert Embankment, London SE1 7TW (020-7339-8500; www.ramblers.org.uk).

Trail Associations offer useful information about specific trails. Once you select a trail, chances are you'll find a website with contact information, managed by a walker's association, to help you.

Walking Britain is the personal effort of Lou Johnson, editor and proprietor. His website, a resource for walkers, provides routes, maps, and descriptions of walks (www.walkingbritain.co.uk).

Public Transportation

BritRail sells tickets and a selection of money-saving rail passes. Many passes can only be purchased outside the UK, so it is best to buy your passes before leaving home. Contact www.britrail.com, or call 1-866-BritRail (1-866-274-87245).

National Rail Enquiry Service offers schedules and advanced reservations. Consult a guide book (suggestions below) for general details about using Britain's convenient rail system. (See Step Four for comments.) Rail prices vary, but are generally less expensive when booked in advance. Contact www.nationalrail.co.uk, www.thetrainline.com, or call 08457-484-950 (24 hours daily) in Britain. In the States, you can call Rail Europe at 877-257-2887 during normal business hours. Be prepared to wait "on hold" for longer than an acceptable amount of time.

Network Express operates an extensive network of coaches (buses). It serves many locations not served by rail. Buses, which are generally slower and cheaper than trains, are often more convenient. For inquiries and bookings, contact www.nationalexpress.com or call 08457-484-950.

Guidebooks

On every path we carry some sort of trail guide. (See Step Eleven, "Trail Guides.") Because "official" national trail guides are quality paperbacks, which can be heavy to carry, we often rely on abbreviated route descriptions coupled with a map or set of maps.

We use other general reference (guide) books as well. They are excellent for trip planning and for sightseeing before or after a walk. For answers to common travel questions, consult one or several of these. Be sure to leave one in your luggage at "base camp." (See Step Four.)

Peruse the travel section of your local book store, or check titles online for books that suit you. A few of our favorits are *Fodor's See It Britain; Insight Guides: England; Let's Go Britain;* and *Rick Steve's England.*

For general walking and planning information, we like *Lonely Planet's Walking in Britain: 52 Great Walks; Walk Britain: The Handbook and Accommodation Guide of the Ramblers' Association;* and *Stilwell's National Trail Companion* (last edition, 2001), which we hope will be updated soon.

General Reading

There are many wonderful books about Britain and British walking. Two of my favorite nonfiction choices—guaranteed to make you smile—are *Brit-Think, Ameri-Think: An Irreverent Guide to Understanding the Great Cultural Ocean That Divides Us* by Jane Walmsley, and *Notes from a Small Island* by Bill Bryson.

To have some fun while polishing your Brit-speak (See Step Eight, "Hard to Say"), peruse the website titled: "(British) English Translated for Americans" (www.uta.fi/FAST/US1/REF/engtran.html).

Good Maps

Good maps are essential take-alongs for a happy walk. Ordnance Survey (ordnancesurvey.co.uk), Great Britain's national mapping agency, sells excellent, detailed maps (at various scales) of the places you'll be exploring. Carrying all the pertinent maps for the entire length of a trail, however, can add significant weight to your pack. (See Step Eleven, "Where Are We?")

Fortunately, some trail associations sell maps for specific paths. My favorite ones are colorful, water-resistant strip maps, which are made by combining relevant portions of the larger maps, along a "strip" of land that forms the route corridor. These are not available for all trails and are best used as supplements to national trail guides and Ordnance Survey maps, especially on a first walk.

Paths Taken

Listed below in alphabetical order are the major paths we've traveled, the approximate mileage covered (the trail, plus the extra miles walked to and from lodging and tourist sites), and a comment about the walk itself. I have assigned each trail a pleasure rating in hiking boots on a scale of one to five, with five being the highest rating. For more information about an individual trail, please see its national trail guide, or contact its trail association, website, or the Ramblers' Association (www.ramblers.org.uk).

Coast to Coast Walk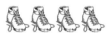

195 (plus 15 extra) miles. St. Bees Head on the Irish Sea to Robin Hood's Bay on the North Sea. Eighteen days of walking, plus a day of rest. (Some walkers do the C-to-C in twelve to fourteen days.) This classic, well-traveled path crosses three national parks. The first (moving west to east) is the Lake District and the most arduous. After this section the track becomes less rigorous. The Coast to Coast Walk was created and first described in 1973 by Alfred Wainwright, a respected fell-walker, whose guide books contain unique, hand-drawn maps and illustrations. The path takes you from the mountains of the Lake District, over the Pennines, through the picturesque Yorkshire Dales, and across the Vale of Mowbray, before it finally traverses the North York Moors. If you are fit and curious, you will love it. It has not yet been made a national trail and could be better waymarked. An experience worth the effort, but not recommended for a first ramble.

Cotswold Way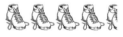

97 (plus 18 extra) miles. Chipping Campden to Bath. Nine days of walking, including one very short day. (Others walk this in six to eight days.) This is a walk through history and some of the prettiest countryside in Britain. Rolling hills, honey-colored stone architecture, stately homes, and quaint villages make the region popular for walking. The Cotswold Way is an especially lovely ramble, although the path can get messy in wet weather.

Dales Way

84 (plus 11 extra) miles. Ilkley to Bowness on Lake Windermere. Nine days. (Many walkers complete the Dales Way in five to seven days.) A popular walk, much of it alongside rivers in two of England's prized national parks: the Yorkshire Dales and the Lake District. It has scenic valleys, green farmland, and moors, divided by rugged stone walls and dotted with charming villages. Pleasant rambling. Few hills. Memorable walk.

Offa's Dyke Path

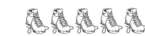

177 (plus 18 extra) miles. Chepstow to Prestatyn. Eighteen days of walking, plus a day of rest. (Some do this in nine to thirteen days.) From the Severn Estuary, this trail travels north along the Welsh border, through the spectacular scenery of the Wye Valley and Shropshire Hills to the Irish Sea. It follows a dyke, or ditch, excavated by the Mercian king, Offa, in the eighth century to keep the Welsh to his west. Today, the path follows about sixty of the eighty miles of King Offa's earthworks that still exist. This well-marked way offers outstanding scenery every day as you walk across high moors, through farmland and dense woodland, and along canal tow paths. Sometimes you walk on the dyke itself. You'll see ancient hillforts, castle ruins, remote villages, and abbeys. Although much of the trail is gentle, its frequent ascents and descents are demanding. Offa's Dyke Path is a wonderful experience, but not an easy walk. Not recommended for a first trek.

Ridgeway

85 (plus 15 extra) miles. Avebury to Aylesbury. Nine days of walking. (Many walk the Ridgeway in six.) Not far from London, it follows a Neolithic trail atop a high chalk ridge, which was in use over 5,000 years ago. The Ridgeway feels like two different walks. The western section, across the Wiltshire and North Wessex Downs, which walkers share with bicycles, horses, and some motorized vehicles, is open, high, rather remote, and relatively flat, with sweeping vistas. The eastern section, in contrast, takes you through the Chiltern Hills and into the villages, woodlands, and farmlands that make this part of the trail so attractive. Not difficult. Very pleasant.

South Downs Way

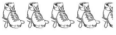

100 (plus 15 extra) miles. Eastbourne to Winchester. Ten days of walking plus a day of rest. (Many walkers complete the SDW in six to eight days.) The trail mostly follows a chalk ridge that provides lovely views. Trails are well drained and not very steep. Walkers share the track with mountain bikes and, in places, horses. Varied scenery. Excellent walk, especially for a first long-distance trek.

Uphill to Old Harry

120 (plus 15 extra) miles. Weston-super-Mare to Swanage. Thirteen days of walking. (Others walk this in eight days.) This patchwork of trails leads from the Bristol Channel southeast across Somerset and Dorset to Old Harry Rocks near Swanage on the English Channel. It wends across classic rural countryside, passing Cheddar Gorge, and entering some of the most captivating communities in England: Wells, Castle Cary, Sherborne, Cerne Abbas, and Corfe Castle. Walkers first follow the nicely waymarked West Mendip Way, before navigating overgrown, lightly waymarked, little-used segments of the Monarch Way and Jubilee Way, finally connecting with the Jurassic Way, which is a national trail. From Lulworth Cove to the sheer cliffs of weathered limestone at Old Harry Rocks, the Jurassic Way walker is treated to an excellent path with spectacular scenery along a steep shoreline trail that hugs chalky cliffs. Except for this section and the areas around villages, few ramblers walk this unofficial route across Somerset and Dorset. Finding and booking B & Bs close to this path is challenging. The route is a good choice for an experienced walker with good navigational skills and a high tolerance for nettles and brambles.

Note: We walked these paths in the order below:
- South Downs Way—April 1996
- Dales Way—September 1997
- Coast to Coast Walk—September 1998
- Cotswold Way—September 1999
- Offa's Dyke Path—September 2003
- Ridgeway—September 2005
- Uphill to Old Harry—September 2007

Frequently Asked Questions

Do You Have a Favorite Path?

Yes, in fact I do. The Offa's Dyke Path. Even with all its ups and downs, it will remain my favorite until I discover a track I love even more!

Are There Many Paths for Walking?

Indeed there are. You'll find about 140,000 miles of public paths in England and Wales alone, including nineteen designated long-distance national trails in the UK. In addition, there are 900,000 hectares (over two million acres) of countryside across which people, according to Natural England, can "walk, ramble, run, explore, climb, and watch wildlife… without having to stay on paths." This so-called "freedom to roam" land of mountain, moor, heath, and down is now delineated on Ordnance Survey maps.

Walkers hold various opinions about how to define a long-distance path. For me, it is a walk of several days totaling fifty miles or more. The Long Distance Walkers Association describes long-distance paths on its website (www.ldwa.org.uk) as walking routes that are twenty miles or more in length, mainly off-road, and generally located in the countryside, although some pass within urban areas, often along green corridors. All this leads one to conclude that the definition of "long-distance" remains in the eye (and foot) of the beholder.

When Is the Best Time of Year to Walk?

People walk in all seasons. We prefer September. Later in the fall, sunset arrives early, and daylight fades fast. In spring, ramblers may encounter less stable weather and walk on wetter paths (although there are many exceptions to any "rule" about weather). In summer, which can be hot, trails and attractions are generally much busier, and pubs and B & Bs fill quickly. Happily, seasonal insects are not a problem, except, perhaps, in Scotland in the spring when the midges hatch.

All this said, the absolute best time to walk is whenever you have the time and can get away.

What Is a Good Distance for a Ramble?

If this is your first walk, a week to ten days is about right. You will want a few days to limber up and to get into the rhythm of a ramble. Once you're "in the groove," you'll be pleased to have several days to relax and enjoy your walk.

For many walkers, this means walking about seventy-five to a hundred miles in total. It assumes that on most days, you'll be walking between eight and twelve miles, perhaps more if you're using a luggage transfer service. (See Step Four, "Principle One: Rate X Time = Distance.")

Decisions about pace, time, and mileage are up to you. Whatever feels right and fits the time you have available is going to be the best choice for you.

IS LUGGAGE TRANSFER AVAILABLE?

Yes. And it can be very helpful. Some services will book your overnight accommodations as well. Many B & Bs also transfer luggage for a set fee if you make arrangements for this when you reserve your room. (See the options described in Step Four.)

Several friends have used luggage transfer services and carried only their day packs. We are thinking about doing this in the future. I have listed below two of the organizations/companies others have found helpful. Check the national trails website (www.nationaltrail.co.uk) to see if there is a luggage service that serves your specific footpath.

• Ramblers' Association: Second Floor, Camelford House, 87-90 Albert Embankment, London SE1 7TW (02973-398-500; www.ramblers.org. uk). For lists of tours and luggage services.
• Sherpa Van Project: 29 The Green, Richmond, North Yorkshire, DL10 4RG, UK (0871-5200124; www.sherpavan.com).

HAVE YOU TAKEN A WALKING TOUR?

I've yet to sign up for a walking tour in Great Britain, although I've enjoyed group travel and some day hiking with organized tours in other locations. For comments on walking tours in Britain and elsewhere, I must rely on friends, who have taken guided and self-guided tours on foot. Our friend Lois, for example, summed up her guided walking tour in the UK this way: "We had an expert local guide for our small, compatible group. We had a van to transfer our luggage, which was also on-call for wet and tired tourists. We stayed in lovely inns and hotels, ate fabulous meals, and, carrying only our day packs, had a worry-free, easy-going adventure in Britain. What's not to like about that?"

All the tour companies my friends like have websites. You can visit them on-line to discover the walking tour that appeals to you. I've listed several of these companies below. You'll find many others on the Web.

- Backroads: 801 Cedar Street, Berkeley, CA 94710
  (800-462-2848; wwww.backroads.com)
- Classic Journeys: 7855 Ivanhoe Avenue, Suite 220, La Jolla,
  CA 92037 (800-200-3887; www.classicjourneys.com)
- Contours Walking Holidays: Gramyre, 3 Berrier Road,
  Greystoke CA11 0UB, UK (017684-80451; www.contours.co.uk)
- Country Walkers: Post Office Box 180, Waterbury, VT 05676
  (800-464-9255; www.countrywalkers.com)
- English Lakeland Ramblers: 15404 Beachview Drive,
  Montclair, VA 22025 (800-724-8801; www.ramblers.com)
- Footscape: 11 Barton Farm, Cerne Abbas, Dorchester,
  Dorset DT2 7LF (01300-341792; www.footscape.co.uk)
- HF Holidays: Imperial House, The Hyde, Edgware Road,
  London NW9 5AL, UK (020-8905-9558; www.hfholidays.co.uk)
- The Wayfarers: 17 Bellevue Avenue, Newport, RI 02840
  (800-249-4620; www.thewayfarers.com)

WHAT ARE YOUR FAVORITE FABRICS AND ITEMS OF CLOTHING?

For each walk, my favorites vary as new materials expand my options. Below I've listed some favorites from my last walk, which I expect to wear on my next one. (See Step Three.)

- Barely There™ underwear (I purchase mine at my local JCPenney department store.)
- Bridgedale™ (Coolmax™) sock liners
- SmartWool™ hiking socks
- Tee shirts made from Coolmax™ or Thermax™ available from many outlets
- Insulating synthetic layers of Capilene™ (light, medium, and expedition weight underwear), available where Patagonia products are sold
- Breathable, lightweight, waterproof, brightly colored rain jacket from L.L.Bean
- All-leather, Cresta Hiker, GORE TEX® backpacking boots from L.L.Bean

Where Do You Shop?

I shop wherever I am when I have some free time. Local stores (not chains) are my favorites. Of course, I also use catalogs and order from outfitters on the Web. To win my heart, my sources must be pleasant about returns, employ knowledgeable sales staff, and maintain reliable stock. I hate learning that an item is out of stock (for the season!) minutes after it appears in a catalog or on a website.

Many fine suppliers exist. I've listed below a few helpful (and probably familiar) vendors to get you started. But first, I suggest that you visit and get to know the folks at your local outdoor "motion" store, where you can sample some good, old-fashioned, in-person attention.

- L.L.Bean: 800-221-4221; www.llbean.com
- Orvis: 800-541-3541; www.orvis.com
- Patagonia: 800-638-6464; www.patagonia.com
- REI (Recreational Equipment, Inc.): 800-426-4840; www.rei.com
- EMS (Eastern Mountain Sports): 888-463-6367; www.ems.com

Why Are Walking Vacations So Popular?

They are an extension of a craze. Everyone who is able seems to be outside walking in all kinds of weather or inside slogging away on a treadmill. People in the United States have embraced "fitness walking" for health, well-being, and as a tool for raising money for good causes.

In Britain, where paths actually lead somewhere and are still used for their original purpose—that is, to take you to a destination—walking is a passion, second only, it appears, to gardening.

Country walking—physically active, low-risk travel—is perfect for a "maturing" population with relatively sound bodies and curious minds. It encourages exploration at a natural pace and entices busy people to relax and tune in to timeless surroundings.

With hundreds of tour operators marketing walking vacations and with trail associations and the Web ready to assist the independent rambler, holidays on foot have become a favorite form of "soft adventure." Their varying degrees of difficulty, their appeal to the active (often older) traveler, and their attractive destinations ensure that these getaways will become even more popular in the future.

Do You Regret Losing Time When Stopping along a Path?

We never think of stopping as a waste of time. There is always a reason to stop. Other than the obvious (resting, drinking, snapping photos, answering nature's call, and eating), cultural and historic attractions literally "stop us dead in our tracks," beckoning us to take a closer look. These include gardens, museums, archaeological sites, historic villages, sweeping vistas across rural landscapes, English Heritage sites (abbeys, castles, country estates, and more), churches and graveyards, giant chalk figures carved into hillsides, hang gliders, and shops selling umbrellas, chocolates, and ice cream.

For us, countryside walking is a vacation, not a forced march. When we walk, we are tourists. And, as tourists, we like to take our time and enjoy the sights.

Afterthought: Step Out

When faced with a decision, some people prefer "making a list and checking it twice." Others are spontaneous and "go with their gut," or intuition. Still others "sleep on it" and see how their decision looks in the morning. Some folks just give up.

Trying to make a decision from beneath today's avalanche of information, I prefer to follow the counsel of St. Jerome, a medieval, biblical scholar. He advised, as did the Romans before him, and Colin Dexter, author of the Inspector Morse mysteries, long after him: *"Solvitur ambulando."* Loosely translated, he is telling us that "the solution comes through walking." Or, as I interpret him, "To solve a problem, take a walk, and the answer will come to you."

May our paths cross often and in fine weather.

Index

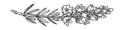

About the Author

A decade ago, Eleanor Berger was a hesitant adventurer who decided to try something new. Reluctant and wary, she gave rambling a try. She has been following footpaths ever since. Now, with more than 1,000 miles under her soles, walking both at home and abroad (mostly in Great Britain), this tenderfoot shares her passion and unique perspective with readers.

The author is an essayist whose personal commentaries have been published in anthologies and magazines, and broadcast on regional public radio stations. She lives with her walking companions—one human, one canine—in northern New York.